MW01485593

P

ENOUGH! ERADICATE BULLYING & INCIVILITY IN HEALTHCARE

Renee Thompson is known internationally as an expert in eliminating bullying and incivility. While Renee has been a nurse for over 25 years, her experience of being a front line nurse leader and educator enables her to speak directly to the heart of critical issues facing the nursing profession today. Not only does Renee include strategies to eradicate bullying and incivility, she includes skills, tools and real-world examples to cultivate a professional, supportive and respectful workforce culture.

Michelle DeLizio Podlesni, RN,
President, National Nurses in Business Association

As someone who focuses on employee engagement in healthcare, I see the negative effects of bullying and incivility. Renee's book is the resource that front line leaders need to address this issue. She provides real-world tools and proven techniques so that managers know how to handle bullies with confidence. Renee tells it like it is. Her content is relatable because she's been in the healthcare leaders' shoes and knows exactly what they are dealing with. Reading this book and implementing the ideas will improve engagement and create a healthy workplace.

Vicki Hess, MS, RN,
Top 5 Healthcare Speaker
author,
6 Shortcuts to Employee Engagement:
Lead & Succeed in a Do-More-with-Less World

Enough! is a fantastic work of practical inspiration that is not only a call to action, but a realistic pathway to addressing the silent epidemic not only in nursing, but in healthcare. Dr. Thompson has once again filled our toolbox with compelling tools for our work as nurses and nurse leaders to turn our caring behaviors on to one another for positive influence and true impact.

Cole Edmonson DNP, RN, FACHE, NEA-BC, FAAN,
Chief Clinical Officer, AMN Healthcare

Enough! is an amazing resource! Renee Thompson has created and proven a formula for putting an end to workplace bullying and incivility in healthcare. In this book, she provides leaders with an unvarnished assessment of this problem, the costs it imposes on healthcare organizations, and the role they must play in building a more positive culture. But Renee doesn't just tell leaders it's their responsibility to fix the problem; she shows them exactly what to do and how to do it. This is the most practical real-world method for addressing disruptive behaviors that I have seen. Every healthcare leader should read this book and then implement the strategies it describes.

Joe Tye,
CEO and Head Coach, Values Coach Inc.

Dr. Renee Thompson uses her knowledge of nurse bullying, combined with lived experiences and a comprehensive understanding of the literature, to find simple solutions to this difficult problem! I love how Renee gives practical tips that any nurse leader can use today. I was so grateful that she even supplied an exhaustive array of complimentary resources that are available in her online "vault." I was especially impressed with the scripting examples for having difficult conversations with nurses. I highly recommend this book for all nurse leaders, regardless of their role or years of experience. Renee and her team really hit the mark with this excellent book.

Perry M Gee, PhD, RN,
Nurse Scientist, Intermountain Healthcare

By sharing true stories and 25+ years of expertise, Renee Thompson teaches leaders to recognize bullying and incivility behaviors, and then gives specific practical strategies to eliminate them. Dr. Thompson provides harsh reminders of this problem we've known about for years but have failed to address and solve. Enough! This book is truly a roadmap for leaders to finally put an end to these insidious behaviors. Armed with the strategies she offers in this book, leaders will be equipped to finally stop the cycle of nurse bullying and incivility. It's about time someone figured out a solution to this problem. Renee Thompson has done just that in this important resource for every healthcare leader.

LeAnn Thieman,
author, Chicken Soup for the Soul for Nurses *series*
and
founder, Self-care for HealthCare™

ENOUGH!

ERADICATE

BULLYING & INCIVILITY

IN HEALTHCARE

Strategies for Front Line Leaders

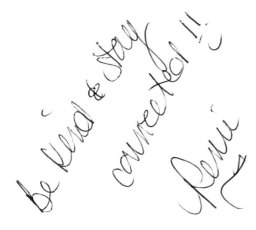

Renee Thompson, DNP, RN, CMSRN, CSP

ENOUGH! ERADICATE BULLYING & INCIVILITY IN HEALTHCARE
STRATEGIES FOR FRONT LINE LEADERS

Disclaimer: This book is intended for general informational purposes only. For legal or psychological advice, consult an appropriate professional.

To contact the author, Renee Thompson, visit
Website .... : HealthyWorkforceInstitute.com
Email .... : WeCare@RTConnections.com
LinkedIn .... : Linkedin.com/in/RTConnections
Facebook ..... : Facebook/RTConnections
Twitter .... : twitter.com/RTConnections
Blog.............. : HealthyWorkforceInstitute.com/blog/

To contact the publisher, inCredible Messages Press, visit
www.inCredibleMessages.com

Printed in the United States of America

ISBN 978-1-7322510-6-9 Paperback

Book Strategist & Editor .... : Bonnie Budzowski
Cover Design .... : Bobbie Fox Fratangelo

To protect confidentiality, names and some details of the stories in this book have been changed.

DEDICATION

This book is dedicated to the front line leaders who know bullying and incivility occur in their departments but don't know what to do about it. This book is for them.

Acknowledgments

When I first started this journey to eradicate bullying and incivility in healthcare, my focus was on individual nurses. As soon as I "opened shop" and proclaimed to the world that enough was enough and that I was taking action against bullying, nurses from all over the world started reaching out for help. For the first few years, I did everything I could to help each individual nurse who shared a personal story about being bullied. I wrote my first book, *"Do No Harm" Applies to Nurses Too! Strategies to Protect and Bully-proof Yourself at Work*, which I dedicated to the thousands of nurses begging for help. I spoke to audiences filled primarily with clinical nurses at the bedside and focused most of my content via blog articles and videos on the individual nurse.

Throughout these years, I noticed a pattern among the numerous conversations I had with nurses. Again and again, nurses told me they had asked their managers for help and the managers "did nothing."

This led me down the rabbit hole into looking at the leader's role in addressing workplace bullying and incivility. Since then, I've shifted my focus toward supporting the leaders who are ultimately responsible for cultivating and sustaining healthy, professional, and respectful workforce cultures by finally addressing bullying and incivility. Since I made the shift, I've talked with thousands of nurse leaders about their struggles to deal with the bad behavior of their employees. Those conversations led me to develop the strategies and tactics you'll find in this book. Without the authentic conversations with leaders, this book would not be possible.

I've worked really hard at becoming an expert on disruptive behaviors. However, doing something with that knowledge and helping leaders requires support and guidance from others.

The good humans in my mastermind groups helped me figure out the focus of this book and have helped me make a bigger dent in the universe: Joe Mull, Kathy Parry, Jeff Tobe, Mj Callaway, Vicki Hess, Denise Ciardello, and Bethanne Kronick. When I'm unsure of myself and feel off track, they boost me up and get me back on the path.

My business coach, Jane Deuber, convinced me that I was no longer a personality company and that I needed to become an institute. She was right. With her guidance and support, the Healthy Workforce Institute was born.

Michelle Podlesni and Louise Jakubik, my sisters from another mother, care enough about me and the success of my business to always give me candid and loving feedback. I'm a better business owner because of them.

My writing coach and cheerleader, Bonnie Budzowski, demonstrated extreme patience with me as I shifted the focus of this book several times, and she still puts up with my fuzzy pronouns. Bonnie helps my words, stories, and strategies make sense.

Without my team of amazing humans, I wouldn't be able to serve as many people: Bobbie Fox Fratangelo, Brenda Violette, Bonnie Artman Fox, Diane Salter, Mitch Kusy, and Cindy DeVore. I'm blessed to be surrounded by them.

My girls, Kaitlin and Courtney, think their mom is "amazing" and brag about me to their friends. Knowing that they are proud of my work is fuel that keeps me going.

Olivia Lauren Hicks, my first grandbaby, fills me with the greatest joy I've ever known. Nonnie loves her dear little nugget!

Lastly, none of this would be possible without my anchor—Ashley, who is extremely comfortable staying behind the scenes (although I do make him come out from time to time), quietly supporting our business and me. Every day on his to-do list, he includes, "Love Renee more."

Contents

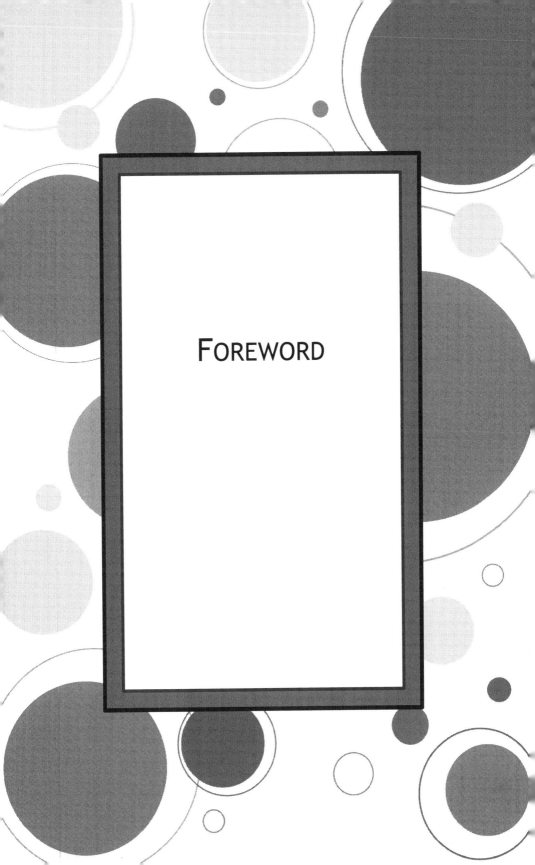

FOREWORD

FOREWORD

In healthcare, we continue to have conversations about bullying and incivility. It's unfortunate and ironic that these behaviors continue to exist in the most caring of professions, nursing.

In conducting research for *Building a Culture of Ownership in Healthcare,* the American Journal of Nursing's award-winning book, which I authored with Joe Tye, we found more than 150 books and articles written on this subject in the nursing literature alone in the past five to seven years. Yet the problem still exists.

With the predictions of huge shortages of healthcare workers in the next few years looming, healthcare leaders must do all they can to create a more positive and healthier workplace environment. Healthcare workers need to be supported in their efforts to provide a safe and quality experience for those entrusted to their care.

The fourth aim of the Quadruple Aim is caring for the caregiver. While nearly every healthcare leader embraces this aim, bullying and incivility still run rampant in our organizations. With over 25 years as a clinical nurse, nurse educator, and nurse executive, Dr. Renee Thompson knows that the problem is not that leaders don't care—it's that they have never been taught how to deal with toxic behaviors. While organizations articulate standards for clinical care and create policies for poor attendance and performance, they do not articulate standards for professional behavior or prescribe disciplinary procedures for uncivil behavior.

Renee Thompson is on a mission to enable healthcare leaders to set behavioral expectations and hold employees accountable for professional behavior. She wants every nurse leader to have the skills and confidence needed to confront and eliminate disruptive behavior. *Enough! Eradicate Bullying & Incivility in Healthcare Strategies for Front Line Leaders* is full of practical, step-by-step strategies for healthcare leaders to create healthy workforce cultures.

I encourage healthcare leaders at every level to read this book.

Bob Dent, DNP, MBA, RN, NEA-BC, CENP, FACHE, FAAN, FAONL
Senior Vice President,
Chief Operating and Chief Nursing Officer
at Midland Memorial Hospital;
2018 President of the
American Organization of Nurse Executives

May, 2019

CHAPTER 1

I DON'T WANT THIS TO HAPPEN TO YOU

What makes the dawn come up like thunder? Courage!

~Cowardly Lion

I DON'T WANT THIS TO HAPPEN TO YOU

On my second day as a front line unit manager, I knew I had made a big mistake in taking the job. The 75 employees I was now in charge of were some of the most unprofessional humans I had ever encountered in healthcare. Nobody had warned me.

In the 14 months I held that job, I went through more stress than I've encountered in my life, before or since. During that time, I left my husband of 18 years and went through what, in retrospect, I consider a nervous breakdown. For 10 years following my decision to quit my job as unit manager, I was sure I was a failure.

I never want you or any other front line leader to experience that level of stress or such feelings of failure.

Here's how I found myself in the unenviable position of accepting that disastrous job: With eight years of nursing under my belt, I loved caring for patients, but my dream of becoming an educator—a teacher—was unfulfilled. I thought about this dream all the time. However, the kind of position I wanted required a master's degree, and I only had an associate's degree. So I enrolled in an RN to MSN program and started my journey to become a nurse educator.

At the time, I was working for a managed care company as a quality director, but I missed the hubbub of an acute care hospital setting. I shared my longing with a colleague who was working as a manager in a large acute care hospital in Pittsburgh. To my delight, my colleague informed me that available educator positions had just posted! I made the assumption that I could start working immediately as an educator, even while going to school.

But, my assumption was wrong. When I inquired about the position, I learned I wasn't yet eligible to work as an educator. I also learned that the hospital had "great front line manager" positions available. Although I had never before considered a management position, I thought such a job could be a stepping-stone toward taking on the role of an educator in the hospital. I thought I could do a great job since I had successfully led a staff of five highly competent, amazing people at the managed care company where I had been working.

I said "yes" to the job of manager without fully understanding what I was saying "yes" to, and my life would never be the same. After I accepted the position, I learned that the unit I was now responsible for had the worst reputation in the entire organization. Did they tell me that during the interview process? Did they say, "In full disclosure, we haven't been able to keep managers longer than a year, and you'd be the sixth manager in six years"? No. I soon found myself stuck, but determined to bring my best to the position.

One morning, the unit secretary asked me to talk with the patient in room 12. The elderly patient had been admitted during the night. She was upset and had asked to speak to the manager. Oh no, I thought. I had learned quickly that my role often included doing damage control following the bad behavior of my staff. What had they done now?

Upon entering this patient's room, I saw a frail and frightened woman. I asked what was wrong, and she explained that the Emergency Department (ED) nurse had tried to alleviate her fears of being admitted by saying, "It will be okay—as long as you don't get admitted to 8B." And there we were in my unit, 8B!

The unit definitely had a reputation, and that reputation was validated almost every day. Here are a few examples:

- One of my nursing assistants who worked nights consistently took a pillow and blanket into the family waiting lounge and napped for an hour or two.

- Another nursing assistant threatened one of my nurses, whom she didn't like, saying that her boyfriend was going to beat the sh** out of her.

- My night shift RN decided to walk off the unit one night to take a cigarette break, even though her patient just went into SVT.

- Some RNs refused to help the LPNs, even during a code situation.

My employees complained to me about their coworkers every day. Each time, I asked them to document the incident so that I could take action, and the response was always the same: "I'm not writing anything down." If they

9

were unwilling to document an incident, I'd suggest that I have a conversation with that employee. But they would beg me not to, "No, no, no, no. Please don't say anything. If she finds out, she'll make my life a living hell." I had never experienced this level of toxicity and fear in any aspect of my life.

Within my first two months on the job, I realized I needed to fire four of my employees. As a leader, I owed this to the human race. Two of these employees were RNs and two were nursing assistants. When I looked into their HR files to see where they were in the disciplinary process, what do you think I found? Nothing. I had to start the disciplinary process from scratch.

After a few months, I decided to look past all that I saw as "bad" and try to figure out the reason why these people—who had chosen to work in healthcare helping others—could behave so badly. I chose to see them as orphaned children going from foster home to foster home, receiving the promise of love, protection, and a commitment to not be abandoned, but then who, year after year, were left by their parent (manager), succumbing to the same pattern: Promise, hope, betrayal . . . promise, hope, betrayal. No wonder they misbehaved!

In my naiveté, I thought these "orphaned" employees just needed love and support. They just needed me to show them that I loved them and that, no matter what, I wasn't going to leave them.

To demonstrate my commitment to my team, I held staff meetings at 7 a.m. and 3 p.m., and often stayed until 11 p.m. to take care of my night staff. Sometimes I came to the hospital in the middle of the night because I wanted them to know I cared about them. I gave out Kudos grano-la bars during the day as I walked through the unit saying, "Kudos to you, and here's a Kudos to you."

I brought in pizza and cookies, and came in on Sundays with my kids, just to say hello. I got the hallways painted and hung pretty pictures to make the environment look better, like a home. I bent over backward for anyone who needed to change his or her schedule, even if it meant that I had to come in and work that person's shift.

I was determined to turn that unit around, and I truly believed I could.

One morning, the night supervisor came into my office, shut the door, sat down, and said, "Renee, I'm really sorry, but I need to tell you something. I was on your unit last night, and your staff members were all sitting at the nurses' station badmouthing you. They talked about how you don't care about them, and how you never hold anybody accountable the way you said you would."

I cried. How could they say I didn't care? I felt that I had sacrificed my family, my friends, and myself to show these people how much I cared. Regarding holding people accountable, all I needed was one more documented incident of disruptive behavior and I could terminate two of my employees. But I couldn't walk around saying, "All I need is one more thing. Give me one more thing and we can get this toxic person off the unit," because it's confidential.

After 14 months, and despite my promise to never leave them, I quit, just like the others did before me. It was a matter of survival.

For years following, I felt that I had not only failed as a leader, but also *was* a failure. Now that I'm older and wiser,

I realize that I never was a failure; I just wasn't equipped with the skills and tools I needed to set behavioral expectations and hold people accountable. Sometimes I wish I could go back and be in charge of that unit again, because now I know what I'm doing.

Once I completed my master's degree in nursing education, I had the opportunity to apply for a corporate position for a large health system where I would basically be responsible for the professional development of over 10,000 nurses. I wasn't sure if I was qualified, but having always been a risk-taker, I took a chance. There was a moment that I almost withdrew my application because I found out that over 100 other nurses had applied for this job!

I immediately questioned whether I was worthy. However, after many layers of interviews, I was selected. The reason, as my boss shared, was because I had experiences in nursing that enabled me to have a 360-degree-view of the delivery of healthcare. I had worked at the bedside, then spent four years in the community as a homecare nurse, then crossed over to the dark side, as many would say, to work for a managed care company. While there, I had performed comprehensive and disease case management and became their quality manager. Then I found myself as the unit manager on that dreadful unit. Knowing how badly I wanted to teach, I had gone back to school, finished my master's degree, and become an educator. No wonder they picked me. I had a plethora of diverse experiences that made me an ideal candidate for the role.

When I look back on each role I held before and after I realized my dream of becoming an educator, I see a consistent pattern. There was always at least one nurse (often more) who seemed secretly to want me to fail. Whether it was the experienced homecare nurse who treated me like I was stupid (until he found out I had a 4.0 GPA and could easily articulate the ins and outs of DIC), the experienced case manager who "forgot" to explain the process for submitting our weekly reports, or the seasoned educator who reluctantly agreed to share her slides with me when I was asked to teach her lecture while she was on vacation—and then placed a passcode on her flash drive (a code she failed to share). Even at the corporate level, my boss seemed to want me to fail when, 10 seconds before I was to present to the chief nursing officers for the entire system, she whispered in my ear, "This is your test. Let's see how good you are." Someone has always tried to squash me.

It wasn't until I was asked to develop new professional development programs for nurses that the stars aligned for me and I began to understand. Throughout this work, I spent a lot of time talking with nurses about what they needed to be successful. Most of the conversations quickly shifted to how badly they were treated by other nurses. This was especially true when I was talking to students and newer nurses.

At the time, I was enrolled in a doctoral program, and I had decided to focus on eliminating bullying and incivility. I just couldn't sit back and say, "Well, that's just the way it is in nursing." I had to do something about it. Since then, I've completed my doctoral program and have become known internationally as an expert in eliminating bullying and incivility. I now know what it takes to address disruptive behaviors in healthcare. I am fully equipped with the skills and tools required to set behavioral expectations and hold people accountable for behavior.

I can't turn back time and undo what happened during my tenure on that highly toxic unit in my first role as front line leader. I can, however, commit to equipping front line leaders with the strategies and tactics they need to cultivate a healthy and professional workforce culture by addressing bullying, incivility, and unprofessional behavior. Together, we can end disruptive behaviors in healthcare.

* * * * *

Imagine a world where nurses are clinically competent and work well as a team; where they go out of their way to support each other; a world where all members of the healthcare team consistently communicate in a respectful manner. Imagine a world where nobody wants to leave because they feel so supported by their coworkers.

Imagine being a leader in this world.

Fairy tale? Well, maybe. But I think it's possible to be far closer to such a reality than we are today. We can move toward practicing kindness and compassion to each other as well as to our patients.

Right now, we often find nurses who are clinically competent but not always nice to each other. Bullying and incivility are alive and well in healthcare, and they are affecting *your* ability as a front line leader to create a healthy work environment.

I know what keeps you up at night:

- You worry about how your employees are treating each other when you're not there.

- You're afraid that the new people you just hired will be eaten alive by your experienced ones.

- You wonder how long you can keep up with the demands your organization is placing on your shoulders because you are spending the majority of your time dealing with bad behavior.

Well, these worries end today!

I never want you to go through the nightmare I went through in my early career. I vow to do everything I can to help you and other front line leaders avoid this.

Over the years, I've learned that creating a healthy work environment *is* possible when leaders are equipped with the essential skills required to set behavioral expectations and hold their employees accountable.

Whether you're a nursing leader in an inpatient or ambulatory care setting or a non-nurse leader in a healthcare setting, that's exactly what you are going to learn in this book. Let's get started.

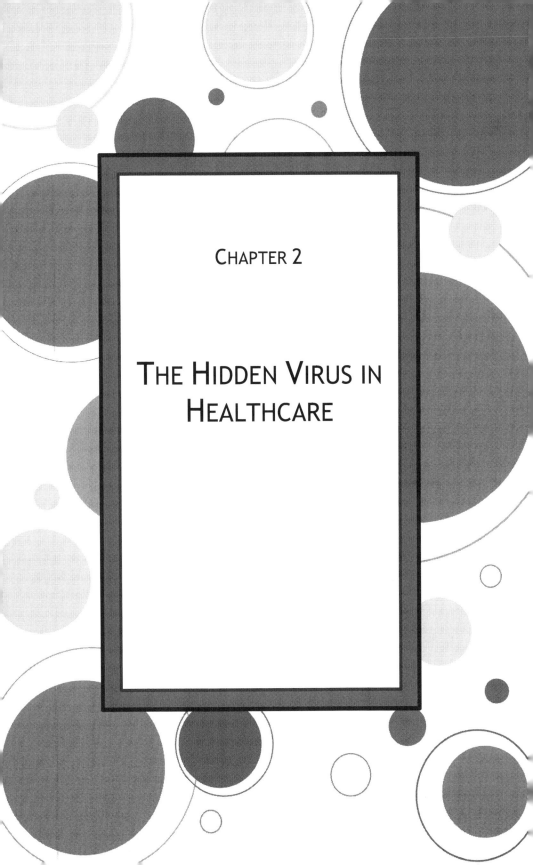

CHAPTER 2

THE HIDDEN VIRUS IN HEALTHCARE

Our prime purpose in this life is to help others. And if you can't help them, at least don't hurt them.

~Dalai Lama

CHAPTER 2

THE HIDDEN VIRUS IN HEALTHCARE

A relatively new nurse, Nancy, was working on a busy med/surg unit known for having the "mean" nurses. They referred to the new nurses as babies, and were clearly eager to see them fail so they could talk about how stupid new nurses were. One day their antics backfired. A 65-year-old patient with a history of diabetes and chronic renal failure was admitted for a non-healing wound to his right thigh. He went to the OR for debridement and blood vessel grafting and then returned to the unit with a Wound VAC. An LPN was assigned to his care; Nancy, with four months' experience was "covering" the LPN. The LPN asked Nancy to come look at the Wound VAC with her because she was concerned.

Together, they assessed the cylinder, which was full of frothy looking blood and agreed that something was not right. Nancy asked for help from one of the experienced RNs, and, after huffing and puffing, she entered the room and said, "Yeah, it's full, change it." About an hour later, the new canister they had placed was full.

Nancy and the LPN consulted the experienced RN again. This time she said, "I'm not holding your hands all day; if it's full, change it." They did what she asked, although this did not feel right. Feeling brave, at least for the moment, Nancy consulted the charge RN. She snapped, "You have bothered Denise about this all day, and there are other patients to take care of. You are like a dog with a bone. Just change it like she told you."

So that's what the two did; they changed it, changed it, and changed it until the patient had a change in mental status, hypotension, and tachycardia. At this point, Nancy notified the manager that they were worried about the patient and could not get help from the experienced RNs. A code was called, but it was too late. The patient died. An autopsy revealed he died from hypovolemia.

Was this an isolated incident, or is this situation far too common in healthcare?

STUDY AFTER STUDY REVEALS A SERIOUS PROBLEM

Numerous studies show the negative impact disruptive behaviors have on individuals, healthcare organizations, and patients. The following study results reflect a sampling— just a sampling—of consequences related to behavior.

The *2016 National Healthcare Retention & RN Staffing Report* by Nursing Solutions, Inc. showed that 70% of nurses reported an association between disruptive behaviors and compromised quality of patient care.

Rosenstein and O'Daniel reported the results of a survey with 4,530 participants. Seventy-one percent said there was a significant association between disruptive behaviors of professionals and medical errors, and 27% believe this link leads to patient mortality.

The Nursing Solutions, Inc. report revealed that 81% of nurses who leave an organization cite peer and nurse-manager relations as a cause for leaving. And the problem is even greater with newly graduated nurses. A study reported in a recent issue of *Policy, Politics & Nursing Practice* reveals that an estimated 17.5% of newly licensed RNs leave their first nursing job within the first year, and one in three (33.5%) leaves within two years.

Townsend reports that of the new nurses who quit their first job within the first six months, 60% state they quit because of the bad behavior of their coworkers. That means that 60% believe culture is more important than a paycheck.

If you're working in an organization where disruptive behaviors go unaddressed, you don't need studies or statistics to validate that bad things happen as a result. You intuitively know this. However, we have the studies to prove it.

DISRUPTIVE BEHAVIOR IMPACTS PATIENTS, HEALTHCARE WORKERS, AND ORGANIZATIONS

Abusive behavior leads to increased stress and decreased concentration, which impacts patient safety. Bullying destroys the team, the collaboration, and any willingness to contribute to a common goal. When employees are uncomfortable communicating with each other, the flow of information stops.

You've probably read or at least heard about the article by the Institute of Medicine (IOM) titled, "Silence Kills." This article clearly demonstrates that when people don't feel comfortable speaking up, patients suffer the consequence.

Healthcare workers pay the price for bullying with their physical, mental, emotional, and spiritual health. Some nurses suffer from PTSD and are no longer able to work because of bullying. Those who manage to work in toxic environments experience decreased motivation and energy at work. And those people take the toxicity home where the impact of extreme stress ranges from irritability to the loss of a woman's menstrual cycle.

A few years ago, I was doing a short, 90-minute workshop on bullying for a group of healthcare employees from different organizations. One nurse, Cindy, sat quietly, seeming to be on the verge of tears the entire time. She stayed after the session and confided in me about a bullying situation that had happened to her.

As Cindy shared her story, she had to stop occasionally to compose herself. Still, she managed to share some horrific experiences she had had with her preceptor. Although Cindy no longer worked with her, she was still petrified at the thought of running into that preceptor somewhere in the hospital. Cindy wouldn't go to the cafeteria or coffee cart for fear that she might see her. When I asked Cindy the last time she had worked with the preceptor, she answered, "Five years!" I could see that Cindy was still traumatized and recommended professional counseling. I felt so bad for her.

Here's how another nurse, Gloria, described the impact that daily bullying had on her:

> I was bullied for two years by multiple people at a hospital where I worked. I didn't recognize that I was experiencing various forms of bullying. I thought it was normal behavior given the high-stress environ-

ment of working in the ICU. I attributed it to alpha personality types and tried to rationalize the behaviors. I even blamed myself.

My self-esteem and ego tanked. I felt alone, insecure, and incompetent. I would often come home after an exhausting 12-hour shift and cry. I dreaded going to work and prayed that I would have a good day. After having to endure this toxic work environment for many months, I developed anxiety and depression. I began to see a psychiatrist that prescribed medication for my symptoms (insomnia, fatigue, moodiness, etc.).

The worst part was that my manager knew what was going on but consistently minimized the abusive behaviors, stated that I needed to get tougher, or turned things back on me. I was alone. After two years, I left.

Make no mistake about it—bullying leaves nasty scars on targets, and time doesn't always make things better.

Organizations pay the price for bullying, literally, through lost profits. Globally, bullying cost organizations over $6 billion per year. How?

As the *Policy, Politics & Nursing Practice* report mentioned earlier indicates, one in three new nurses leave their jobs within the first two years, mostly because of peer and nurse-manager relations. Another study indicates that when bullying is present, 45% of nurses leave their unit and 34% leave their organization. The cost of turnover is astronomical, but the costs don't end there. I've talked with many nurses who look at their schedule before getting ready for work. If they see they are working with the queen bully, they call off. Then the manager has to spend time trying to fill that hole, sometimes using an agency or incurring overtime costs.

A 2018 study conducted by RNnetwork revealed that 49% of respondents have considered leaving the nursing profession in the last two years.

"The fact that half [of nurses] are considering leaving their profession should be a wake-up call for the healthcare industry," said Lynne Gross, vice president at RNnetwork. "These survey findings reveal areas where providers can work together with nurses to improve working hours, reduce instances of workplace bullying and harassment, and address mental health."

Despite the numerous studies validating that bullying and incivility are the causes of turnover, related costs, and poor patient outcomes, they are allowed to continue. A study by the Workplace Bully Institute indicates that only 6% of healthcare leaders have identified eliminating bullying and incivility as a top priority. Ninety percent say bullying and incivility are problems in their organization. Why aren't healthcare leaders making eliminating disruptive behaviors their number one priority?

We need to do a better job!

ENOUGH IS ENOUGH

The good news is that bullying and incivility in healthcare are finally getting attention from regulatory agencies. In April of 2018, The Joint Commission (TJC) released a Sentinel Event Alert that includes shocking statistics about workplace violence in healthcare and recommendations for organizations to act.

Let's look at a few definitions of workplace violence:

Violent acts (including physical assaults and threats of assaults) directed toward persons at work or on duty.

CDC National Institute for
Occupational Safety and Health (NIOSH)

An action (verbal, written, or physical aggression), which is intended to control or cause, or is capable of causing, death or serious bodily injury to oneself or others, or damage to property. Workplace violence includes abusive behavior toward authority, intimidating or harassing behavior, and threats.

U.S. Department of Labor

In October of 2017, The Magnet® Recognition program added criteria for Magnet® designation regarding addressing physical and verbal violence. EP15EO requires organizations seeking Magnet® designation to show robust data and interventions regarding workplace violence, bullying, and incivility toward nurses.

The American Nurses Association (ANA) gathered expert nurses to discuss and develop a position statement regarding disruptive behaviors. In 2015, the ANA released a position statement on bullying, incivility, and workplace violence. In their statement, they include intervention recommendations for employers and employees.

While these recommendations and requirements provide organizations with "what to do," they don't get to the root of how to stop the tsunami of disruptive and dangerous behaviors.

I heard a story about an executive leader who hosted a mandatory meeting with all the organization's front line leaders, 80 in total. During this meeting, the executive shared results from recent surveys that showed high turnover due to bullying and incivility. He told everyone at that meeting, "Starting today, you're going to start holding your employees accountable for their behavior. Go take care of it," and then he left the meeting.

If you had been one of the 80 leaders in that meeting, my guess is that you would have felt frustrated, even angry, at the executive's behavior. As a front line leader, you hate toxic behaviors and cultures as much—even more—than anyone else. You are the ones spending inordinate amounts of time dealing with the impact of toxic behaviors and cultures. If you knew how to stop it, you would.

As you might have predicted, two years after the executive's charge, that organization reached out to me for help because nothing had changed. They were still losing good people because of bullying.

It's unfair to say, "Start holding your people accountable" without teaching leaders *how* to actually do that. That's my job and my passion. I teach leaders how to take the recommendations from the regulatory agencies, the study outcomes, and the generalizations that we get regarding leadership, and take them down to action at the department level. I answer the questions: What do you say? When do you say it?

We are hemorrhaging nurses, providers, and support staff to bullying and incivility and putting our patients at risk. Organizations, therefore, need to do a better job equipping front line leaders with the skills and tools they need to cultivate a healthy, professional, and supportive workforce by eradicating workplace bullying and incivility.

A culture of silence must be replaced by a culture of safety.

I know that you, as a front line leader, want practical strategies that you can adopt immediately. By the end of this book, you will have the tools, strategies, and confidence to identify disruptive behaviors that undermine a culture of safety, set behavioral expectations with employees, and hold staff accountable for professional behavior.

I'm so glad you're here. Are you ready?

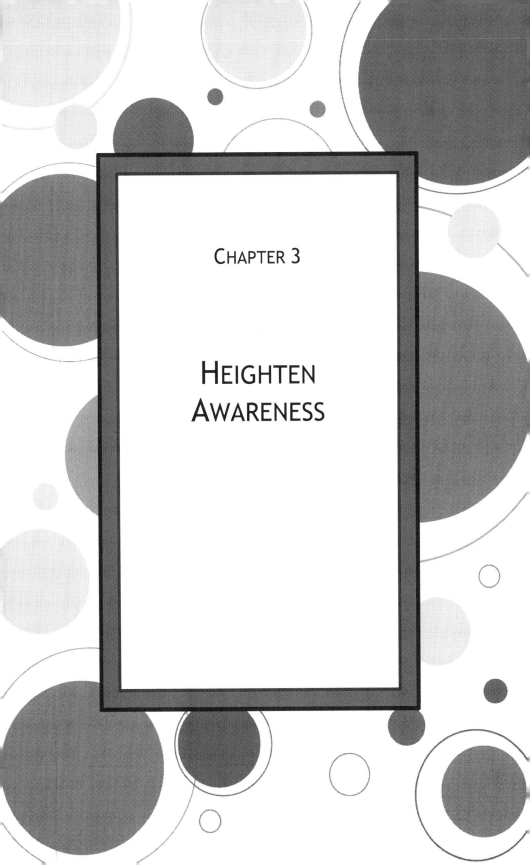

CHAPTER 3

HEIGHTEN
AWARENESS

Awareness is like the sun. When it shines on things, they are transformed.

~Thich Nhat Hanh

Chapter 3

Heighten Awareness

Aparticipant in my online course, *Eradicating Bullying & Incivility: Essential Skill for Healthcare Leaders,* wrote the following comments on her course evaluation:

> When I was signed up for this course I thought, "Oh great. Why do I need to take this? We don't have bullying in my workplace anyway." Boy, was I wrong. When I started paying attention, I saw it [bullying and incivility] almost every day.

When I talked with this participant during a one-on-one coaching session, she shared that in 29 years of nursing, she had become numb to the eye rolling, condescending attitudes, nitpicking, and even overt criticism, cursing, yelling, gossiping, and mocking in her workplace. She just stopped noticing it.

This competent and caring individual had *normalized* the deviance in her healthcare setting.

You've heard the classic illustration: If you drop a frog into boiling water, the frog will jump out. But if you drop a frog into tepid water and slowly increase the temperature to boiling, the frog will sit there until it boils to death. The frog dies from a deadly situation it can easily escape—but only if it *recognizes* its environment has become toxic.

Coming to work in a healthcare environment can be like getting dropped into tepid water. Awareness of your environment is essential to your health—sometimes even your survival.

How do know if you or others have normalized disruptive behaviors in your organization? If you hear any of the following statements regarding someone's behavior in your workplace, you are in tepid and rapidly heating water:

- Well, that's just the way she is. Don't let anything she says bother you. Don't take it personally.

- If you have any questions, don't go to him. He doesn't like people very much.

- You're going to have to grow a thick skin if you want to survive here.

We've accepted bad behaviors to the point where we fail to recognize them as abnormal. It's time to take the temperature of our environment. For example,

- A 2012 study showed that 21% of novice nurses report they are exposed to bullying behavior daily.

- A recent Occupational Safety and Health Administration (OSHA) survey reports that over 50% of registered nurses and nursing students have been verbally abused (a category that included bullying) over a 12-month period.

Numerous studies show the prevalence and devastating impact disruptive behaviors have on retention, patient safety, and the financial health of the organization, yet few top healthcare executives are paying attention. (You'll remember a recent study cited earlier that indicates that only 6% of top healthcare executives named eliminating disruptive behaviors as a top priority.)

Are they guilty of the boiled frog phenomenon too?

I once listened to a discussion about bullying and incivility during an advisory board meeting with healthcare leaders. One chief nurse executive said, "Oh, we have no bullying in my organization." Really? I knew for a fact that she did because some of her nurses were asking me for help.

Isn't it time we un-normalize deviant behavior?

If you're reading this, you probably already know your department has an issue with disruptive behaviors. However, if you're like most leaders, you may not be quantifying the problem in any meaningful way. You know you're tired of the complaining, the drama, the fighting among your staff, and the he said/she said conversations you have with your employees, yet you don't know where to start to fix the problem. Tackling disruptive behaviors within your department can feel like an overwhelming challenge. When feeling overwhelmed, many of us do what's comfortable—we avoid the problem and do nothing.

Doing nothing ends today! In the next several chapters, I will walk you through a step-by-step process for transforming your workforce culture in a way that goes beyond telling your employees to get along and just be nice to each other. The process starts with heightening awareness.

Following are the three primary strategies to raise awareness of bullying, incivility, and even workplace violence:

1. Assess your current culture by quantifying the types and frequency of disruptive behaviors happening in your department.

2. Engage in honest conversations with your employees.

3. Start on the path toward educating and training your employees so that they (and you) can gain clarity on what bullying is; what it's not; how disruptive behaviors show up in the workplace; and what they and you can do about it.

Once you go through this process, not only will you show up differently, but over time, so will your employees!

Assess Your Current Culture

After reviewing the results from exit surveys, one of my clients discovered that 50% of his new nurses were quitting because of bullying and incivility in their critical care units. That data prompted him to hire me to conduct a comprehensive assessment in his organization, which validated the results from the organizational exit surveys and uncovered what was really happening on those units. Armed with that information and some guidance from me, my client was able to take action to stop the bullying behavior. Now the turnover rate in those departments is 10%.

Before you can solve a problem, you need to fully understand the problem. Therefore, assessing and understanding your current culture is the first step in heightening awareness of disruptive behaviors.

The process of assessing your current culture is similar to conducting an admission assessment like nurses do when admitting patients. Sometimes, when we ask a patient if he's had surgery, he answers "no." When we lift up the gown, however, we find a road map!

"Oh, that scar was my appendix ... and that's from having my gallbladder removed." While many bedside nurses dread these long admission assessments, they're critical to the overall care of the patient. Before long, nurses learn that to deliver appropriate, individualized care to patients, they must first lift the gown.

Assessing for bullying and incivility is no different.

To eradicate bullying, you first need to lift the gown to discover what's underneath—what's happening, how prevalent, how often, where, and to whom disruptive behaviors are happening. Thankfully, there are several assessment options to choose from.

Using Surveys to Assess Culture

I once ran across a statistic indicating that 40% of all targets of bullying don't speak up. My experience tells me the statistic is reasonably accurate. When employees are dealing with disruptive behaviors from their coworkers, they may be reluctant to tell anyone out of fear of retaliation, reprimand, or because they don't want to appear weak. This is especially true when the target is a new employee. Frequently, employees within your department who witness the behaviors won't tell you either. As the manager with a myriad of responsibilities, you may have no idea.

Conducting surveys enables you to find out what's happening in a non-threatening, confidential, and anonymous manner. Surveys can identify specific disruptive behaviors and quantify their frequency. Surveys enable you to gather data that can serve as baseline metrics to show positive outcomes after you've implemented any interventions.

Another benefit of conducting a department survey is that it sends a message to your employees that you value their input, you want their feedback, and that their experiences beyond their clinical work matter.

Surveys can be conducted at the organizational level, and you can use them to tease out specific results related to behavior. However, the very best way to find out what's happening in your department is to conduct a departmental survey.

Department Level Surveys

One of the easiest and best ways to find out what's happening in your department is to conduct an anonymous, confidential, disruptive behavior survey. These surveys can be conducted electronically or via old-fashioned paper and pen.

Hard copy surveys may be necessary if you currently have a strained relationship with your employees. When conducting a comprehensive assessment with a large healthcare organization, we found we had to use old-fashioned paper and pen because there was so much mistrust between the employees and the leadership team. When the organization tried to conduct any electronic survey with their employees, they had less than a 5% response rate! Why? Because the employees thought their leaders had a super-secret way of knowing who answered each survey. That's the level of distrust that was present between employees and their leaders in the organization.

If something similar is true in your organization or department, don't beat yourself up over it. Simply seek to know where you are starting, even if it means you're starting at the bottom.

When I'm asked to conduct a comprehensive assessment in an organization, or when I'm starting my department deep dive consulting, we always start with my Disruptive Behavior Assessment. This assessment includes 15 questions using a 5-point Likert scale and categorizes the responses into witnessed and experienced.

Over the last eight years using this assessment, I've discovered that the results will always indicate a higher number of witnessed incidents of disruptive behaviors versus ones that are experienced. This validates the notion that more employees are witnesses to bad behavior than targets of it. Unfortunately, most witnesses neither stand up to the bully nor report him or her.

In my Disruptive Behavior Survey, I have specific questions regarding common bullying and incivility behaviors, which include the following:

- Being yelled at, criticized, or cursed at in front of others
- Receiving an uneven workload assignment, seemingly based on favoritism
- Being excluded by certain nurses from routine lunches and celebratory or social events
- Having accomplishments downplayed, such as awards or advanced degrees
- Being ignored or given the silent treatment by certain nurses

- Being treated nicely to your face but mocked or insulted behind your back

Analyzing results from a survey like this will allow you to discover what some of the most common behaviors are within your department. Then you'll have a better understanding of where you need to focus. For example, if your department scores high on "Receiving an uneven workload assignment, seemingly based on favoritism," you need to evaluate how your charge nurses or coordinators are making assignments.

Once you establish your baseline data, it's important to reassess every six months so that you can show a decrease in disruptive behaviors in your department.

To download a complimentary copy of the Disruptive Behavior Survey, go to https://theHealthyWorkforceInstitute.com/Resource-Vault/

Organizational Surveys

If, however, you want to start with data already conducted by your organization, or you're an executive leader wanting to conduct an organization-wide assessment, there are a few survey options healthcare organizations use.

Most healthcare organizations conduct surveys with their employees. These surveys commonly assess employee engagement, employee satisfaction, cause for turnover, and employee morale. This data can shine a light on behavioral issues, providing data for further assessment and analysis.

A number of survey companies are popular in healthcare. Press Ganey, Gallup, The Advisory Board, and PeoplePulse™ are the big four. These companies do not assess behaviors specific to bullying or incivility. Their surveys are usually more about teamwork, employee engagement, or the relationship with their manager. However, some of the questions included in an organizational survey can suggest issues regarding behavior, which can then be further evaluated.

For example, in the Gallup Q12 Survey, question five asks, "Does your supervisor or someone at work seem to care about you as a person?" If your employees score low on this question, it may provide you with a clue that relationships among employees are strained, which could be related to disruptive behaviors.

If you choose to start your assessment by looking at your existing data results from an organizational survey, look for any questions that focus on relationships. If bullying and incivility are prevalent in your department, you should expect lower scores on relationship and communication questions.

Surveys Specific to Disruptive Behavior

A few surveys specific to incidents of disruptive behavior are available. However, it's rare to find an organization that utilizes them.

The Negative Acts Questionnaire

The Bergen Bullying Research Group of the University of Bergen in Norway created a comprehensive questionnaire to determine the presence of bullying behavior. The Negative Acts Questionnaire was created specifically to determine behaviors without using the term bullying in order to guide participants in answering questions more accurately on the basis of the behavior rather than the behavior's label.

Nurse Incivility Scale (NIS)

This scale was created using focus groups of 163 hospitals surveyed to identify nurses' incivility experiences stemming from various members in the hospital hierarchy, using a priori scale construction. It's very effective for use in hospitals and nursing environments.

Focus Groups

During a focus group with over 25 new nurses (which is higher than the ideal size), I noticed a young female nurse, Katie, sitting in the back of the room. She either looked completely disinterested or she was really struggling with my questions about how she and her colleagues were being treated as new nurses. I seriously couldn't tell.

I paid attention to Katie as the meeting ended, and sure enough, she remained in her seat. Once everyone had left, Katie asked if she could speak to me privately, but she could barely get any words out. Immediately, she started to cry. Katie shared a few examples of how the other nurses treated her and was trying to figure out if she should quit or just toughen up and stick it out. After all, she was working in the ICU, and it was only her second week on the job. Katie was hoping things would get better but was losing hope.

Here's one example that highlights the level of cruelty she experienced: One day, Katie's preceptor had to step off the unit. She asked Katie to prepare medications for a critically ill patient. When the preceptor returned, they would give the medications together.

While Katie was preparing the medications, she had a question about one of them and wanted to call the pharmacist. Since Katie didn't know the number for the pharmacy, she approached one of the nurses sitting at the nurses' station and asked for the number. The nurse replied, "Sure. It's 1-800–go f*** yourself!" Katie was shocked, not only because of his response to her, but because some of the other employees sitting at the nurses' station just sat there and laughed. No one made an attempt to help Katie find the number.

The unit manager had no idea this was happening even though she had met with Katie on several occasions to see how things were going. Katie never mentioned her struggles with coworkers.

I've learned that people, especially those on the receiving end of disruptive behaviors, typically won't talk to their administrators about it—but they'll talk to me. Bringing in an outside expert to gather input from employees is an excellent way to find out what's happening on the ground level.

I've learned more about what's actually happening in my client organizations than any of the surveys those organizations conduct. Why? Because employees share everything with an outsider! Without reliable information, a leader may be trying to fix the wrong problem!

One hospital asked me to conduct my comprehensive assessment because they believed their biggest issue was with their older, more experienced nurses. What I discovered during the focus group validated their concerns, but it also uncovered another major issue that they didn't know about.

I discovered a surprising depth of bullying by some of their charge nurses. On one unit, if the charge nurse liked you, she gave you the easier patients. If she didn't, you got the worst, most complicated patients. Some nurses figured this out. If they knew this charge nurse was working, they would call during the time she would be making assignments and play dumb, "Oh. I didn't know you were working today..." and then offer to "stop by Starbucks" to bring her favorite coffee. These nurses resorted to bribing their charge nurse just to get an easier assignment.

I've heard stories like these repeatedly, and when I share the stories with the leaders, they are often shocked and frequently admit that they had no idea what was going on. They just knew they had a problem.

Conducting focus groups can provide you with the intelligence of what's really happening in your department.

Be a Fly on the Wall

To ensure you haven't normalized deviance on your unit, start paying attention to your employees by standing back and simply observing, like a fly on a wall! You'll be amazed at what you see and hear.

Look out for the following types of statements:

- You've got to pay your dues.

- It's always been done this way.

- I'm making her a stronger nurse.

- If she thinks I'm hard on her, wait till she meets _____.

- Just suck it up, buttercup.

- It's sink or swim here, so if you want to survive, you'd better learn how to swim.

- Just ignore him like everyone else does.

> HWF BEST PRACTICE TIP
>
> PAYING ATTENTION
>
> Shelby Smith, a nurse leader in my course, *Eradicating Bullying & Incivility: Essential Skills for Healthcare Leaders,* has a great habit of paying attention. Rather than answering emails in her office, she checks email in the nurses' station or somewhere else in the department where she can observe her staff. Shelby sets up her computer at the nurses' station once a day for an hour to go through emails. This enables her to get caught up on her emails while quietly observing her employees. She catches a lot of behaviors, professional and unprofessional, that she would otherwise miss if she weren't consistently present.

I suggest that you spend time observing your employees during common times when we tend to see more disruptive behaviors:

- During shift reports
- When the charge nurse has to assign a new admission
- During bedside rounds with the providers

Just pay attention. You'll be amazed at what you see!

ENGAGE IN HONEST CONVERSATIONS WITH YOUR EMPLOYEES

I met Brenda when I was asked to conduct a workshop at her hospital. She approached me after the program and asked for advice. Actually, Brenda spent the first five minutes complaining about her employees—how mean they were to each other; how they constantly complained to her about each other; and how nitpicky and condescending they were to new employees and anyone who got pulled to her unit. Brenda praised her team members' level of clinical competence, but she was disgusted with how they treated each other, "They are so great with our patients, but they're so mean to each other!"

Brenda talked non-stop until I gently interrupted her with a question. I asked, "Have you ever told your team members exactly what you are telling me? Have you ever had an honest conversation with your team members about their behavior?"

She stopped talking and looked at me as if I were speaking a foreign language. It had never occurred to Brenda to be honest with her employees.

As leaders, we must engage in honest conversations with employees if we are ever going to decrease incidents of disruptive behaviors. Don't assume your team members are aware that you notice both their clinical competence and their cruelty toward each other. It's your responsibility to tell them.

Engaging in honest conversations with your employees not only raises awareness of disruptive behaviors, it also helps prepare them for the work ahead. Honest conversations about current unit culture and behaviors can heighten awareness of how they are treating each other and how their behavior impacts the work, the patients, and each other. Awareness is the first step in un-normalizing disruptive behaviors.

Start by scheduling a meeting with your employees. You might choose a previously scheduled staff meeting, a time after a hospital-wide training when you know many of your employees will be present, or an ad hoc meeting. Let your employees know ahead of time that the purpose of the meeting is to talk about a healthy workforce initiative you plan to implement in your department.

Begin this meeting by stating your intent. For example, "My intent for this meeting is for us to have an honest conversation about our department, how we treat each other, and the opportunity we have to make our department a great place to work." You want your staff to view this initiative as an opportunity to create a more professional, supportive, and nurturing workplace.

Say something positive (if it's true) about the department first:

- *We give great clinical care to our patients.*

- *In a crisis situation, you all respond in a way that gives me pride in our work here.*

- *The clinical skills on this unit are among the best in the hospital.*

The key is to let them know what they do well as a team. Then let them know what they need to work on.

Use key phrases/statements:

- *This is a professional environment, yet we have not been treating each other and the people who support us in a professional manner.*

- *The way we've been treating each other is not okay.*

- *We have an opportunity to create a more professional, supportive, and nurturing environment.*

- *It's an expectation that you get involved and do your part.*

- *I would be concerned if anyone WOULDN'T want to get involved.*

Avoid negative language such as the following:

- *Our unit is so bad that we have to do an intervention.*

- *Bullying and incivility won't be tolerated any more.*

- *We have the worst department in the hospital.*

- *The way you treat each other is terrible.*

The key in this step is to engage in conversations with your employees as a group (I'll teach you how to have honest conversations with individuals in Chapter 4). This meeting is all about heightening their awareness of how they treat each other. Trust me, when they walk out of the meeting, not only will they start paying attention to how their coworkers treat each other, but they will also pay attention to their own behavior.

As the leader, it's your job to create the vision of what your department can look like, what it can become. But you have to be honest about where you are right now.

EDUCATE AND TRAIN YOUR EMPLOYEES

I've been conducting workshops on addressing disruptive behaviors for almost 10 years. After my workshops, many attendees stay to personally thank me, ask for specific advice, or just share a comment. One of my favorite comments was from an executive leader who said, "We had a wound we didn't know we had. A nice Band-Aid covered the wound we didn't know was there. You came in, ripped off the Band-Aid, and exposed the wound!"

After you've had the initial honest conversation with your employees, it's important that you start talking about specific behaviors that contribute to an unhealthy work environment so you can, in a sense, expose the wound.

In my experience, one of the biggest areas of confusion that makes it difficult to eliminate bullying and incivility is misunderstanding about the differences between bullying, incivility, conflict, and someone just having a bad day. Therefore, an important step to educating and training yourself and your employees is to get clear on what bullying is and what bullying is not.

Employees often complain to their boss that they're being bullied. They may say things like, "Tina is such a bully. I hate working with her!" If you don't fully understand what actually constitutes bullying, you can easily get sucked into the vortex of drama. Many times when employees complain about being bullied, the behavior in question is not bullying at all.

How do you know if your employee is a bully, or perhaps just a drama queen, or a jerk? How do you know if your employee is just having a bad day?

Although there isn't a national legal definition of bullying in the United States, most experts, like myself, accept the following as the definition: Bullying is repeated patterns of disruptive behavior with the conscious (I know I'm doing this to you) or unconscious (I'm not even aware) attempt to do harm.

For a behavior to be considered bullying, there needs to be three components:

1. A Target
   There has to be a target. This target can be a single person or a group of people. For example, someone might pick on just one new nurse and make her life a living hell while being nice to everyone else. Group targets can include the opposite shift (a nurse on days who hates all nurses on nights), new nurses, or support staff who have a particular ethnic or geographical background.

2. Harmful
   The behavior has to be harmful in some way. This harm can be to the target (I have a visceral reaction every time I have to work with this person) or harmful to a patient (a nurse who sabotages or sets a nurse up for failure, affecting patient care).

3. Repeated
   I believe this is one of the most important elements of bullying. The behavior can't be just a one-time event (I scream at you during a crisis). The harmful behavior has to be repeated over time. Some experts say six months or more constitutes a pattern of bullying. I disagree. I consider a behavior as bullying if it's repeated several times over the course of a few weeks. For example, think about orientation.

A few examples will make the distinctions clearer.

I recently had a nurse reach out to me who insisted that his organization was bullying him. When I asked for specifics, he said that his organization was forcing him to wear a mask because he wasn't willing to get the flu vaccine. I asked whether or not he was the only one being forced to wear a mask. Of course he said "No," that anyone who refused the flu vaccine had to wear a mask.

Is the organization bullying this nurse?

No. The organization is unilaterally enforcing a policy based on evidence-based practice!

Terri and Bonnie usually get along. However, today they got into a heated discussion about assignments. Bonnie was in charge and made a decision to assign Terri a more complicated new patient instead of her stable patient from the day before. Terri was the most experienced nurse on staff that day and Bonnie made the decision based on what she thought was best for the patient. However, Terri didn't see it that way. Terri accused Bonnie of babying the newer nurses and dumping on her. The discussion ended when Terri grabbed Bonnie by the arm and yelled, "I'm so tired of this crap!" as she stormed past her.

Is Terri a bully?

No. Terri committed a single act of aggression, which needs to be addressed, but it's not bullying.

Every time Camelia followed Chad, she refused to take report from him. Once she made the comment, "Trust me. There's nothing you can tell me that I can't find out for myself." Despite your insistence as leader that she take report for the sake of the patients, Camelia refused to take report from Chad. However, you noticed that she takes report from everyone else.

Is Camelia bullying Chad?

Yes! We can clearly see that she's targeted Chad (takes report from everyone else), the behavior is harmful (to patient care), and it's been repeated over time.

This is bullying.

I do a lot of deep dives in organizations. As I mentioned earlier, I pull back the covers and lift up the gown. You'd be surprised what I find. Actually, I don't find a lot of bullying among employees. But I do find an awful lot of incivility.

Incivility Is Different than Bullying

Incivility is both different from bullying, and way more pervasive. While the behaviors can be similar, they tend to differ in intensity. Incivility shows up as rude or inconsiderate behaviors. It's the eye rolling, the condescending treatment, the favoritism, gossip, or mocking.

The American Nurses Association does a nice job defining incivility: Incivility is one or more rude, discourteous, or disrespectful actions that may or may not have a negative intent behind them.

For example, someone cuts in front of you while you've been waiting in line forever; a cashier ignores you when you say hello; or a coworker uses the last piece of paper in the printer but doesn't fill the tray— incivility is rampant in the world.

While one-quarter of the people surveyed in 1998 reported being treated rudely at work at least once a week, that figure rose to 55% in 2011 and 62% in 2016, according to Christine Porath, author of *Mastering Civility: A Manifesto for the Workplace.*

Another survey, called Civility in America 2016, found that 74% of the 1,005 US adults questioned believed civility has declined in the past few years. A whopping 70% say incivility has risen to crisis levels.

In healthcare, incivility can be just as damaging as bullying. Why? Because managers are more likely to ignore uncivil acts than they are true bullying behaviors. However, make no mistake about it: incivility is a killer to a healthy and professional workplace!

A study conducted by the Institute for Safe Medication Practices (ISMP) regarding peer-to-peer and interdisciplinary incivility questioned participants regarding the following behaviors with the following results:

- Negative comments about colleagues or leaders—encountered by 73% at least once, by 20% often

- Reluctance or refusal to answer questions or return calls—77% at least once, 13% often

- Condescending language or demeaning comments or insults—68% at least once, 15% often

- Impatience with questions or hanging up the phone—69% at least once, 10% often

- Reluctance to follow safety practices or work collaboratively—66% at least once, 13% often

Almost half of the respondents said intimidation altered the way they handle order clarification and questions about medications.

Here are other examples of incivility from nurses:

Leah was a new graduate in a nursing residency program who worked on a floor where the nurse educator was disrespectful. The nurse educator talked down to Leah, rolled her eyes, and made rude comments to her in front of other nurses. Leah wanted to approach the nurse educator but was afraid it would negatively affect her work life. Leah was questioning whether or not becoming a nurse was a good decision. She was considering leaving the profession.

Tanya worked on an L&D unit where there were a lot of new nurses. She was a seasoned RN and had difficulties with the younger staff of new nurses that were running amok with mean-spirited behavior that was not being addressed by management. They were quick to criticize others, sigh, and roll their eyes when told their patient needed something. Instead of serving patients, they would sit at the nurses' station talking about their social lives while the support staff ran around caring for *their* patients. Tanya had noticed that other nurses who spoke up were retaliated against. She had gone to HR only to be told it's just "girl drama" and to deal with it. Tanya was depressed to the point where she hated thinking of going to work and got anxious before starting her shift. She was actively looking for other positions.

Incivility can show up as rude and obnoxious comments about others:

- A med/surg nurse is pulled to an ICU. The charge nurse takes one look at her, rolls her eyes, and says, "They sent us *this*? Why bother?"

- A charge nurse calls a young nurse a "slacker" in front of a group of her peers when she states that she is having difficulty with her patient assignment.

These behaviors are unlikely to meet the definition of bullying, yet it's easy to see the negative impact they have on the individual nurse, the nursing profession, and the organization.

SIMPLE INCIVILITY TEST

You get into your car, which is parked in a busy parking lot at the grocery store. While putting on your seat belt, you notice that someone is waiting for your spot.

Do you hurry up and put your seat belt on so you can give them your spot quickly?

Or do you take your good ol' sweet time and let them wait? *Which choice do you make?*

What Bullying Is *Not*

Constructive Criticism
When an employee receives constructive criticism from a preceptor, more experienced nurse, or the manager, it is not bullying! Yet, so many nurses claim that they're being bullied because someone was honest with them about their behavior or practice.

The Manager Holding Staff
Accountable for Performance

Many nurses complain that their boss is bullying them because they were put on corrective action for not following policy, not coming into work on time, calling off too many times, not giving medications, telling a coworker to "kiss my **s," etc. This is *not* bullying! It is being held accountable for your nursing practice.

A nurse reached out to me for help with a bullying boss. Her exact words were, "My boss is bullying me." Now, sometimes the boss *is* the bully. According to the Workplace Bullying Institute, 64% of all bullies are in a supervisory role. Still, it's better not to make assumptions. I asked this nurse, "What did your boss do to make you think she was bullying you?"

"My boss wrote me up," she answered.

I asked, "What did your boss write you up for?"

"For calling off," she replied.

"How many times did you call off?" I asked.

"Fifty-seven," she replied! (Well, I'm exaggerating a bit. It was about 13 times.)

That's not bullying!

When a boss is trying to hold the employee accountable for his or her performance, it is *not* bullying! However, employees are quick to pull the bullying card.

Conflict and/or Expressing a Different Opinion

Just because you have a conflict or disagreement with a coworker or your boss doesn't mean either of you are bullies. Conflict is different. Conflict is *not* bullying.

Having a Bad Day
and Getting "Testy" with Your Coworkers

Let's face it. Nurses work in stressful environments filled with unpredictability and complexity, and we are not always on our best behavior. I challenge you to claim that you've *never* done or said anything unprofessional at work when under stress. It's a human thing. This does not make us bullies!

Let's all get clear on bullying versus everything else. Once we do, we can focus our efforts on stopping the cycle of bullying, which has *no* place in a profession dedicated to caring and compassion.

> HWF BEST PRACTICE TIP
>
> BULLIED OR SOMETHING ELSE?
>
> Dr. Cole Edmonson, a former CNO, shared that when one of his employees tells him he or she is being bullied, he replies, "Okay. I believe you. Now let's unpack this." He then listens to his employee's story and evaluates whether or not the employee is truly being bullied or if it's something else. As the leader, it's important that YOU understand the difference so that you can educate your employees.

Bullying and incivility are alive and well in healthcare, yet we're hopping around like boiling frogs, ignorant to our surroundings. If you're not doing anything about this in your organization, not only are you putting your patients and employees at risk, but you're also in violation of regulatory requirements. Make a commitment starting today that you will no longer just accept bad behavior as the norm and that you'll take action by heightening awareness.

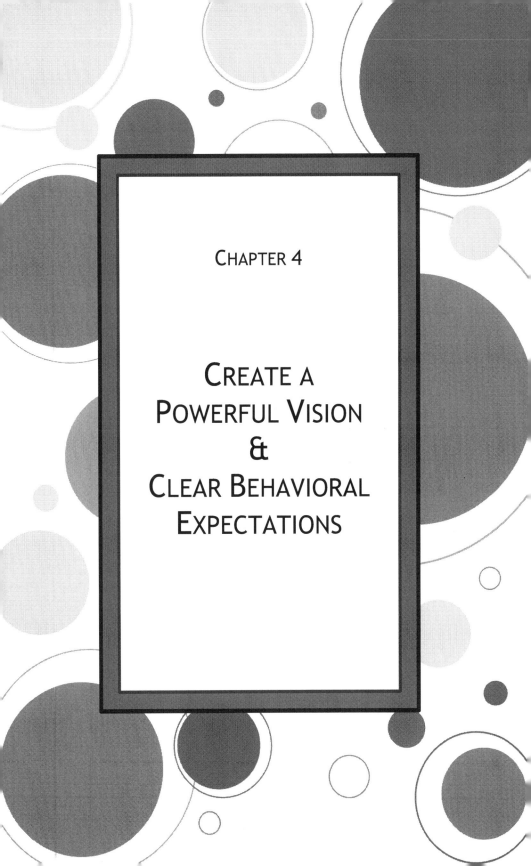

CHAPTER 4

CREATE A
POWERFUL VISION
&
CLEAR BEHAVIORAL
EXPECTATIONS

"Would you tell me, please, which way I ought to go from here?" asked Alice.

"That depends a good deal on where you want to get to," said the Cat.

"I don't much care where," said Alice.

"Then it doesn't matter which way you go," said the Cat.

~Alice in Wonderland

CHAPTER 4

CREATE A POWERFUL VISION
& CLEAR BEHAVIORAL EXPECTATIONS

Functioning as an adult didn't come easy for me at first. I married young and had two kids right away, without the means to provide for them. We survived on food stamps, government cheese, and peanut butter. One day, when looking into an empty refrigerator and then at my hungry kids, I felt a "flip of the switch" in my brain. I realized I wasn't living the life I had thought I was going to have. In that moment, I knew that nobody was going to save me, and if I wanted a better life for my kids and myself, I needed to take 100% responsibility. The first thing I did was think about the type of life I wanted. I created a vision for my ideal life.

At first, my vision was simple—food for my kids and money to pay my bills. Over the years, my vision expanded to owning a home, getting advanced degrees, being in a loving relationship, and starting my own company.

I put myself through school, worked really hard, and never gave up or made excuses for what I had or didn't have. I just kept focusing on a vision of what could be.

For decades, owning a winter home in Florida was one of my goals, and I recently bought that home. The first time I stood in my new bedroom overlooking the water after signing the last new homeowner document, I was overwhelmed with emotion because I clearly remembered what it was like when I had nothing. I remembered dreaming about the type of life I wanted, and there I was, living it.

In any situation in which you desire a change, you first need to determine where you're going. Then, you need directions on how to get there.

In Chapter 1, I asked you to imagine a world where nurses are clinically competent and work well as a team; where they go out of their way to support each other; a world where all members of the healthcare team consistently communicate in a respectful manner. This is a world nobody wants to leave because everyone feels so supported by coworkers. Did you find yourself imagining what it would be like to be the leader in that world? What if I told you it can happen?

You *can* create this world, but first you need to get very clear about your vision, especially about the type of culture you want for your department—for your employees. In Stephen Covey's, *7 Habits of Highly Effective People*, Habit #2 is: Begin with the end in mind. Starting here is important because the vision of what could be (the end) determines the path you need to take along the way.

In this chapter, we'll explore:

- How to create a vision of what your department could look like

- The positive direction the military can offer healthcare

- How to turn your team into a wolf pack (yes—wolves)

- The importance of establishing clear behavioral expectations

- How to involve your team in setting behavioral expectations

CREATE A VISION FOR YOUR DEPARTMENT

Take some time to imagine what you want your department to look like in one year, five years, and ten years. Be specific. What do you want others to say about your team? How do you want your employees to show up every day? What do you want to *feel* when you arrive at work each day?

As you develop your vision, be sure to review your organization's documents regarding its mission, vision, values, any codes of conduct, and any policies related to employee behavior.

Review everything to get an understanding of your organization's expectations for employees. The worst thing you can do is to create a vision and expectations that are misaligned with those of your organization. You'll want to incorporate the same or similar language in your department's vision and expectations.

In my company, I have both a mission statement and a vision statement. Many people get confused between the two. I was confused too, until my curiosity forced me to explore the differences.

A mission statement is written in the present (current state). It's the reason for your existence. A vision statement is written in the future, what could be (desired end state). For example, my mission statement for the Healthy Workforce Institute is as follows:

Our mission is to eradicate bullying and incivility in healthcare.

This statement reflects our core business, what we currently do. Our vision statement looks like this:

Our vision is to be known as the leading experts in the field of workplace bullying and incivility within the healthcare industry.

Although we are the only company that focuses on eradicating bullying and incivility exclusively in healthcare, we haven't yet penetrated the entire market. Not every healthcare organization knows about us. Our vision creates a future world where all healthcare organizations immediately think of the Healthy Workforce Institute when they need solutions to their disruptive behavior problems. We're on the path but not quite there yet. Having the vision keeps us on track, the way GPS does when we travel to support our clients.

Here are a few examples of mission and vision statements in healthcare departments:

Post-Anesthesia Care Unit (PACU)

Our mission is to recover patients from anesthesia safely, then efficiently transfer them to the next level of care.

Our vision is to create a healthy environment for employees and a healing environment for the patients recovering from surgery.

Medical Intensive Care Unit (MICU)

Our mission is to deliver the best possible care to patients in crisis and restore their health as quickly and safely as possible.

Our vision is to set the standard for how care is delivered to critically-ill patients.

Mother-Baby Unit

Our mission is to provide the highest quality, safe, and compassionate care to moms and their newborn babies.

Our vision is to make our unit a place where we care just as much for each other as we do for moms, dads, and their precious babies.

As the leader, you determine the vision for the culture you want to create. Once you're clear on where you're going, you can lead your team there.

When I think about cultures in healthcare, two unlikely metaphors come to mind for such a caring profession: the military and wolf packs! Let's start with the way military decision-making can inform good healthcare practice.

POSITIVE DIRECTION
FOR HEALTHCARE—FROM THE MILITARY

Consider the following passage from a *Harvard Business Review* article about teamwork in the military:

> After dinner at the Quantico officers' club, a Marine general explains to the MBA students that in combat a commander must unequivocally commit to two objectives: (1) Accomplish the mission; and (2) Bring all your people back from the battlefield, whatever their condition. Mission first, then team, then self.

A military mission is a coordinated effort by teams made up of individuals, all working together to accomplish that given mission. The mission always comes first. The team mission is second in that it takes a team to accomplish most missions. Individuals in the team must also focus and train on accomplishing not only the team mission, but the overall mission, putting self-interest aside.

It's a simple formula: Mission first, then team, then self.

In healthcare, we are inclined to have it backward. I see a lot of employees making decisions based on what's best for them, not their patients, and certainly not their team.

This was clearly the case for Karen, a nurse on a cardiac step-down unit. As far as the charge nurse could tell, Karen's goal when she came to work each day was to avoid getting an admission.

Karen did everything possible to delay transferring her patient to the next level of care until 30 minutes before the end of her shifts.

The charge nurse constantly reminded Karen that she needed to move her patients so that she could admit postop patients who were waiting for a bed. Karen gave excuse after excuse: "The bed's not ready; I tried to give report but the nurse was at lunch; the family wants the patient to stay for a little while longer;" and more.

One day, after getting a litany of Karen's excuses, the charge nurse actually walked up to the receiving unit and found that the bed in question had been ready for hours. The receiving nurse had never gotten a call from Karen. Busted!

In *The Fifth Discipline*, Peter Senge talks about alignment, noting that when everyone is making decisions based on one primary goal (the mission), work takes less energy and things get done faster. However, when everyone is running amok, doing his or her own thing based on individual goals (self), both energy and time are wasted.

Think about the time, energy, and frustration the charge nurse wasted trying to get Karen to transfer her patient—time and energy she could have used to care for her own patients (she had an assignment too!). Think about the impact of Karen's behavior on her coworkers on the unit. With her attitude, it's doubtful that she was helping other members on her team manage their challenges. Think about those patients in the recovery room who were waiting for a bed. Think about the stress on the family members who were waiting to see those patients.

If I went to your department today and asked your employees to articulate their goals, as well as the mission of your unit, I would probably get a dozen or more answers. For some nurses, the goal might be to get everything done on their task list. For others, it might be to care for patients as if they were precious family members. But as you know, for a few nurses, the goal is to do the least amount of work possible, get the easiest patients, and avoid any new admissions!

I bet you have a few Karens in your department.

In my workshops, I ask participants to make a list of behaviors they consider disruptive, ones that they've either witnessed or experienced. Any time I see behaviors on the following list, I know that people are focusing on themselves rather than patients or the team:

- Hides when there is a crisis (otherwise known as ghosting)
- Demonstrates lack of teamwork
- Dumps work on others
- Claims "that's not my job," etc.

Whether participants in the workshops are employees or leaders, *lazy* always makes the list. (Of course, lazy isn't actually a behavior, but the behaviors listed above point to an overall attribute of laziness.)

Think about the impact to your team and your patients when you have employees who are perceived as being lazy. Who on your team is making decisions based on what is best for self?

Perhaps the problem of laziness and other assorted disruptive behaviors lies in faulty decision-making. Perhaps we can teach our teams how the military makes decisions.

Mission First

What's your mission? How does your mission show up every day? Do your employees incorporate the mission into their conversations, or are they going from task to task?

As we talked about earlier, creating a compelling mission and vision is an important step to cultivating a healthy workforce. If your employees aren't clear on what the mission is, they will make up their own missions.

Your department needs a mission—something that drives decision-making. When I work with organizations to create professional and supportive work environments, one of the activities we do is to create a mission/mantra statement.

Team Second

Nurses tend to get myopic when it comes to their work: my patients—my shift—my unit—my organization. They fail to see how everything they do or don't do has a trickle-down effect on everyone else, thereby affecting the mission too.

What happens when a nurse focuses only on self? Examples include the nurse who retimes all her medications for the next shift so she doesn't have to deal with them and the Karens who hang onto their patients so they don't have to get an admission. Think about how that selfish behavior impacts everyone else on the team. It does.

During my tenure as a clinical instructor, I would take a group of students onto a unit. On our first day together, I would tell them that when they were done with their work, before they were allowed to sit down, they had to check with every other student to see if he or she needed help. Then, they had to check with every nurse on the unit, and then they had to check with the support staff. Only when they had offered to help everyone on the unit could they take a break.

Team—then self. One way a leader can reinforce "team second" is by adopting a "Before-you-leave checklist." On that checklist is an item that every employee needs to answer before leaving the unit: Check on your colleagues before you leave—are they okay? As the leader, you need to do the same.

Before you leave for the day, connect with all employees to see if they are okay before you walk off the unit. After all, they are your colleagues, too.

> HWF BEST PRACTICE TIP
>
> CHECK IN AND CHECK OUT
>
> One of the managers in my *Eradicating Bullying & Incivility* course adopted a "Check in and check out" strategy. As soon as he arrived on the unit, he would "check in" with every employee present on the unit. Before he left, he did the exact same thing. The employees grew to expect and look forward to his "check ins" and "check outs" because they all knew he wouldn't sneak in or out without letting them know.

Self Third

Nursing is a service profession. By the nature of the job, we are inconvenienced every day we walk into work. Think about it. We should be in the habit of making decisions based on what's best for the patients, not ourselves. Once, when I was working as a professional nurse at the bedside, the coordinator on duty apologized because she had to give me an admission. I said, "That's what I'm here for, to get admissions."

To be honest, my inside voice said, "Crap. I have to get an admission!" I had just gotten caught up and didn't feel like getting a new patient. However, like it or not, taking care of patients was my job—and it deserved priority over my needs. Self should be last.

A nursing director, Sasha, told me a story of how she explained this concept to an employee, Carla, who was upset after getting floated to another unit for two days in a row. Carla was angry and said it was hard to keep working in the department after getting passed up for charge nurse two different times and then getting floated two days in a row.

Sasha explained, "We work together as a department and we float to where the patients' need is the greatest, because patients come first." She affirmed that Carla was a great nurse and takes great care of *her* patients. However, Carla didn't consider the needs of her peers or other patients on the unit. Sasha talked about the importance of putting patients first, our peers next, and ourselves after that. She let Carla know that once she could put her peers and their needs ahead of her own, they could start looking at a charge role. First, Carla needed to not only prove she is a team player but also show her peers she cares for them and supports them in their roles as well.

Another concept in the military makes good sense in healthcare: Mission first, people always.

It's difficult to accomplish the mission when your people are distracted, unmotivated, or motivated by the wrong things. A leader must know how to take care of his or her people so they can complete the mission. If a team member is toxic, having issues at home, or is ill, that team member needs to be taken care of so he or she can help the team complete the mission. And, of course, none of us can do our job well if we don't take care of ourselves. Getting enough sleep, eating well, and exercising are all vital ways to care for ourselves, enabling us to complete our mission.

HWF BEST PRACTICE TIP

REINFORCE A TEAM MINDSET

During huddles, staff meetings, and the start of each shift, recite positive affirmations that reinforce a team mindset, like they do in the military. Here are some to choose from:

- *We may have all come from different ships, but we're all in the same boat now. ~Martin Luther King, Jr.*

- *What do we live for; if it is not to make life less difficult for each other? ~Mary Ann Evans*

- *Individually, we are one drop. Together, we are an ocean. ~Ryunosuke Satoro*

- *The cumulative effects of our everyday choices have the power to transform the world. ~Kelly Coyne, Erik Knutzen*

- *Coming together is a beginning; keeping together is progress; working together is success. ~Henry Ford*

- *It is one of the most beautiful compensations of this life that no man can sincerely try to help another without helping himself. ~Ralph Waldo Emerson*

- *If you want to lift yourself up, lift up someone else. ~Booker T. Washington*

- *Let us be kinder to one another. ~Aldous Huxley's last words*

- *Our work is not just about getting tasks done. It's also about making a difference in the lives of our patients and each other. ~Renee Thompson*

The military structure is a good reminder of the priorities we need to have in healthcare. Another metaphor that makes sense to me is likening nurses to a pack of wolves—in a positive way.

HOW TO TURN YOUR TEAM INTO A WOLF PACK

According to Twyman Towery's *The Wisdom of Wolves*, these animals are more devoted and committed to their family and community than any other mammal on earth. Nothing will stop a wolf, not even the threat of harm or death, from protecting the pack. Each pack member takes full responsibility for supporting and protecting every pack member, no matter what.

Imagine if nurses behaved this way—protecting their pack above all else. That would mean that every new nurse would be nurtured, supported, and protected from harm, and every patient and family member would be included in the pack. Every nurse then would take full responsibility for all patients, and all nurses would go out of their way to ensure the success of their coworkers.

Several years ago, I was fortunate to get a glimpse of what working with a wolf pack might be like when I was working casual status as a bedside nurse. I was teamed with another nurse and her student in a five-bed step-down unit. In this mini unit, we didn't have a nursing assistant, so we had to rely on each other. Throughout the day, I was amazed by the pack behavior of this nurse and her student.

Here are a few examples of how they demonstrated wolf pack behavior:

- I had a patient in isolation that needed to be repositioned and cleaned. I asked for help but then my other patient needed to be medicated for pain. I told my coworkers to give me a minute to take care of my patient in pain; however, as soon as I treated my patient, I saw that they were already gowned and gloved, in my patient's room, taking care of her. Done!

- The student told me my patient was incontinent (all over the bed). I immediately asked if she could help me (the patient was obese), but she said she and the other nurse had already taken care of it. Done!

- The student walked another patient to the bathroom—twice, which was not an easy thing to do because of the two IV poles, a catheter, and NG Tube.

- I was getting a transfer from the med/surg unit. Not only did my team members help me get the patient settled, a coworker also noticed the patient's medications were due and gave them for me! Done! (Don't worry, she asked me first.)

I have no idea how I would have been able to care for the patients assigned to me the way I would want my family to be cared for if it hadn't been for these amazing nurses.

What can you do to create wolf pack-like behavior in your unit or department?

Adopt a Wolf-Pack Mindset
A wolf pack mentality is that of extreme loyalty and devotion to the group, which binds them together as a unit, despite times of hardships and stress.

Coach K, Mike Krzyewski, who has been honored as one of the greatest college basketball coaches, once said, "The goal is to create a dominant team where all five fingers fit together in a powerful fist." The ability to care for patients effectively, compassionately, and safely requires that everyone sees himself or herself as part of the same hand, as one team with one goal.

Put the Performance of the Team First—Not the Individuals

Wolves are highly social animals that live in packs. A pack is an extended family group comprised of different skills, strengths, and weaknesses. However, as a pack, there isn't any group stronger.

When I worked on a cardiac unit, I was really good at drawing blood gases but not so good at managing chest tubes (still hate them). As a cohesive team, we all knew the strengths and weaknesses of every other nurse on the team. When *any* patient on the unit was ordered a blood gas, whoever was assigned that patient asked me to draw it (if I was working). If I had a chest tube, some of the other nurses knew to stop by periodically and check my system (bubbling okay here but not there!). We all knew that for our patients to receive the very best care, they needed the skills and strengths of all of us, not just the nurse they were assigned to that shift.

In healthcare, our overall mission should focus on providing extraordinary care to patients and their families. It is the decisions employees make every day that determine how well that happens.

THE IMPORTANCE OF
ESTABLISHING CLEAR BEHAVIORAL EXPECTATIONS

One day, as my husband and I were walking out of a pharmacy, he said, "Hey, Renee, I've noticed that sometimes you are disrespectful to cashiers."

I replied, "What are you talking about?"

He said, "Just now, when you went to pay with a credit card and the store didn't have a self-swipe unit, you just put your credit card on the counter."

I said, "Instead of what?"

He responded, "Instead of handing the card to the cashier, and I've seen you do the same thing before." He had noticed a pattern of behavior in me.

I said, "Whoa, whoa, whoa. You mean to tell me that when I put my card on the counter instead of handing it to the cashier, you think it's disrespectful?"

He said, "Yes, I do. It's like you don't even have the courtesy of handing your card to the cashier."

Since this exchange with my husband years ago, I've asked hundreds of people in my audiences to raise their hand if they also think it's disrespectful to put your credit card on the counter instead of handing it to the cashier. Roughly 30-40% raise their hands.

Since the initial exchange with my husband, every time I shop in a store that doesn't have a self-swipe credit card unit, I ask the cashier, "When people pay with a credit card, do you find it disrespectful if they put their card on the counter rather than handing it to you?" Guess how many of them have viewed it as disrespectful? Roughly 95%.

I strive to be one of the most respectful humans on earth; I teach respect, yet I was being disrespectful and didn't even realize it. I knew that the behaviors of greeting a cashier, smiling, and thanking the person for his or her help were respectful. I was unaware that the behavior of setting my credit card on the counter instead of in the cashier's hand was disrespectful. I needed my husband to point this out in a clear and specific way. In doing so, he prompted me to set a behavioral expectation for myself.

In healthcare, we do a really good job setting expectations when it comes to clinical care. We tell nurses to give medications on time, document patient education, follow CORE measures, and adhere to regulatory requirements, etc. However, we do a lousy job setting behavioral expectations beyond coming in to work on time and not calling off (or in).

When it comes to how to behave as professionals and treat people, we are far less specific. We tend to give people a code of conduct to sign during orientation and assume that takes care of it. I once had a human resource director argue with me about the importance of getting employees to sign their code of conduct. He insisted that all employees should continue to sign their code upon hire and told me I was wrong for suggesting otherwise. I leaned in, looked him in the eye and said, "If signing a piece of paper changed behavior, then why did you call me for help?" Asking employees to sign a piece of paper may be a good start, but it's not enough.

Setting behavioral expectations is just as important as setting clinical expectations. If you've never done this before, talking to your employees about how they should behave might feel uncomfortable. You might be thinking that you shouldn't have to tell adults how to behave in a professional environment.

The reality is that if left on their own and without structure, even adults can run amok—especially when under pressure. This is why it's important that *you* believe telling your staff exactly how you expect them to behave is essential. If you believe it, they will too.

* * * * *

A new adjunct instructor in an RN-BSN program grading her first writing assignment wasn't prepared for the attacks she received from her students. As an instructor, it was important to her to explain why she took off points and what students could have done differently to receive a better grade. Sometimes, it would take her over an hour to grade a three-page paper because she spent so much time providing feedback.

Even so, some of her students argued with her, citing that she wasn't clear in her instructions and that's why they didn't meet expectations. If she didn't include in the instructions, "The interview must be conducted with a leader who works in healthcare," even though most of the questions were about relationships among disciplines on the *healthcare team*, how could she take off points?

So, the instructor revised the instructions to be clearer. Yet, students still found a way to argue that she wasn't clear enough.

So, she created a rubric. Still not clear enough.

She created a rubric and included examples from previous students who got it right (names removed of course).

Until finally, her instructions were so clear that a toddler could have aced the assignment!

It may sound like the instructor was too accommodating to her students by allowing them to defend their grade. The truth is, she was still learning how to be an instructor and questioned her competence from time to time.

Once the instructor got crystal clear on the instructions, it was so much easier for her to stand firm on her decision when a student argued about a grade.

I know you have employees who always seem to find a way to turn any blame back to you! I also know that sometimes you blame yourself, or at least question yourself.

Setting clear behavioral expectations makes it much easier for you to stand firm when you have to counsel an employee about his or her behavior.

Let's say, for example, you're the manager in the emergency department (ED) and the expectation (priority) is to move patients from point A to B. Every one of your employees needs to work together to move the patients through triage, treatment room, and then onto the next level of care. By communicating that moving patients through the ED from point of entry to final destination is the expectation, all employees know exactly what role they need to play regarding flow.

This example is about process and workflow. You can communicate similar expectations regarding behavior. Let's say you suspect or even know that when other staff gets pulled to your unit, they are not always treated professionally. You can clearly set the expectation that any time someone gets floated to your unit or is from an agency, that person automatically gets the easier assignments, first dibs on meal breaks, and that the person in charge will touch base with that individual throughout the shift. Once you clearly communicate that this is an expectation, nobody has to think about what to do when a float or agency nurse arrives. Everyone should be on the same page, like it or not.

By setting the expectations up front, it's much easier to identify when expectations haven't been met. Let's say you find out that someone was pulled to your unit and given all of the isolation patients. Now you can engage in a conversation with the charge nurse about how expectations were not met. And, when discipline is necessary, clear expectations pave the way for an easier process.

Unclear expectations are one of the most common sources of frustration for employees. When they don't know what's expected of them but are then criticized or disciplined when they don't meet those fuzzy expectations, employees become disgruntled and disengaged. I've talked to many nurses who complain that their manager changes his or her mind frequently and they never know what they are supposed to do.

To minimize this frustration and lack of clarity, it's important that you prepare to set both clinical and behavioral expectations. The question isn't whether you should or shouldn't set expectations. The question is what and how?

Christina Hernandez, a director of surgical services, provides a good example of setting clear expectations. Six years ago, when she stepped into the director role, Christina identified issues regarding following policy and process, a general lack of accountability from her staff, and disrespect among the team. Since then, she's completely transformed her department. Her strategy was to make sure everyone was clear with regards to both clinical care and the way they treated each other.

Christina, a participant in my *Eradicating Bullying & Incivility* course, shared an example during our coaching call of how she engages her employees in conversations about failing to meet expectations. These conversations resulted in her employees actually giving her permission to discipline them!

When an error is made, she asks to meet with the employee in her office. Christina informs the employee of the issue and then asks the employee these questions:

- *Do we have a policy (or process) for this ___?* The employee answers *"yes."*

- *Can you walk me through the policy/process steps?* She does this to make sure the employee actually knows the correct policy.

- *Did you follow this policy/process?* At that point, the employee recognizes he or she violated the policy and is much more receptive to counseling and, if necessary, disciplinary action.

Christina keeps the employee in her office until one of two things happen: the employee thanks her or laughs.

You can do the same with behavioral expectations once you've set them.

How to Involve Your Team in Setting Behavioral Expectations

Experts agree that success rates of organizational change initiatives are abysmally low. Beer and Nohria set the failure rate at 70%. Why? It's because organizations don't involve their people in the change process from the beginning. When you don't involve your employees, the transformation you're trying to achieve becomes your project—not theirs.

Although employees don't have input on the mission, vision, and strategic goals of their organization, they do and should have input on the mission, vision, and strategic goals within their department.

First, schedule a staff meeting with your employees. Let them know that the purpose for the meeting is to determine, as a department, expectations they have of each other as a team. Give them the heads up that you will be asking them to come to the meeting prepared to discuss ways they always want to be treated by each other and ways they never want to be treated by each other.

Second, during the meeting, place four pieces of easel paper on the wall. At the top of each, write one of the following headings:

Disrespectful (on 2)   **Respectful (on 2)**

Start the meeting by sharing your vision to cultivate a respectful, nurturing, and supportive environment. Where everyone goes out of their way to support each other—where everyone makes decisions based on what's best for patients and each other. Although your organization has established values and a code of conduct, you want your team to develop their own.

Equally important is to define the behaviors that *do not* represent respect and support, such as cursing, criticizing in front of others, ignoring a call light from a patient that isn't yours, etc.

Ask the group to think about the behaviors they've experienced at work and what category they fall into: disrespectful or respectful.

Ask them to write down a specific behavior on a sticky note that they believe contributes to a respectful work environment and then place that sticky on the "respectful" board.

Then ask them to write down a specific behavior on a sticky that they believe violates a respectful work environment and to place that sticky on the "disrespectful" board.

Some examples may include the following:

Disrespectful
- Yelling at someone in front of others

- Talking about someone behind his or her back

- Cursing

Respectful
- Saying good morning to a coworker while smiling

- Talking to each other directly when there is a problem

- Helping each other with patient care

Optional:
Once the group has populated each category, ask them to each choose three disrespectful behaviors they *never* want to experience by placing a colored dot sticker next to them.

Then ask them to select three respectful behaviors they *always* want to experience by placing a colored dot sticker next to them.

Collate the answers and use them to develop a unit-based professional practice agreement, which you will post on the Healthy Workforce Bulletin Board (see Chapter 7 for instructions). Here are some tips to help you facilitate the discussion:

- Encourage staff to list 10 behaviors for each category. You may need to give them some examples to stimulate ideas.

- Remind them to write only one behavior per sticky note.

- Sometimes employees will write behaviors that are too vague. For example, "negative attitude." If you see this, ask the question, "What does negative attitude look like? Can you be more specific?"

Note: Any behavior that may potentially impact patients holds a higher weight.

Make sure you leave the boards on the walls for one week to allow other employees who were not able to attend the meeting the time and opportunity to contribute. Also, as people think about behaviors, they may add to the boards as the week progresses. Let everyone know you'll leave the boards up for one week and encourage continued participation.

Once you're satisfied with the input from your employees, collate the behaviors listed on the board by looking for common themes. Take those themes and then craft them into a draft professional practice agreement.

Once you've crafted your draft agreement, make sure you give a copy to every employee. Give them one week to provide any feedback and then finalize your agreement, give everyone a fresh copy, and post your agreement on your Healthy Workforce Bulletin Board.

Review this agreement with your employees every six months and make revisions as needed.

To download the "Always and Never" activity and receive a few examples of professional practice agreements, go to https://theHealthyWorkforceInstitute.com/Resource-Vault

By getting the employees to identify the behaviors you want and the behaviors you don't want, you increase their intrinsic motivation to maintain and enforce the expectations. You determine the overall goal of a healthy workforce culture; let your employees determine the process of getting there.

When all employees can articulate the expected goals and behaviors, you can hold them accountable.

The leader must help employees function with an understanding that they are part of something greater than themselves. A belief in the mission is critical for any team or organization to cultivate a healthy workforce. It's a bit easier to do this in healthcare because our mission generally involves patients. Use this to your advantage and sprinkle reminders everywhere.

You're the leader. You're the "captain of the ship." You determine the direction you want your ship to go. Equipped with the strategies laid out for you in the next few chapters, you'll be able to navigate through the storms and rough waters along your journey.

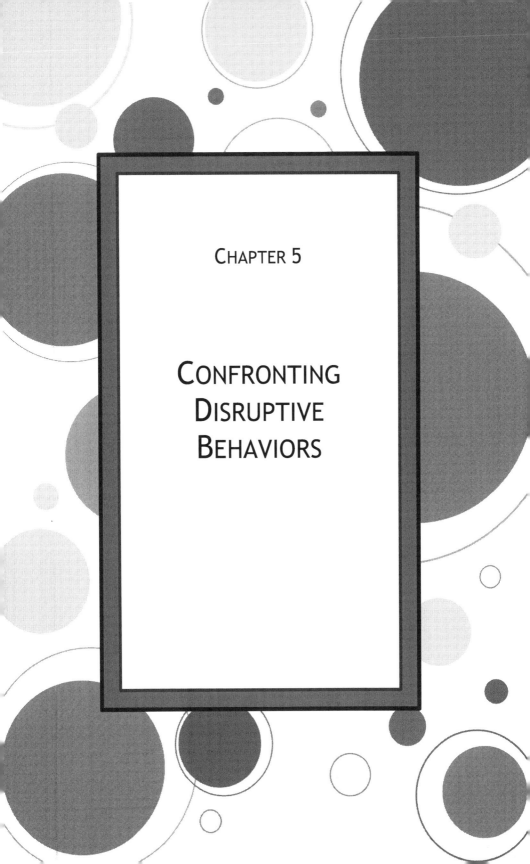

CHAPTER 5

CONFRONTING
DISRUPTIVE
BEHAVIORS

In any moment of decision, the best thing you can do is the right thing, the next best thing is the wrong thing, and the worst thing you can do is nothing.

~Theodore Roosevelt

CHAPTER 5

CONFRONTING DISRUPTIVE BEHAVIORS

During the interview process for the disastrous unit manager position I've told you about, I was asked to meet with the staff. I remember sitting in a conference room facing a few of the nurses, nursing assistants, and one unit secretary. A question that kept coming up throughout our conversation was, "Are you going to hold people accountable?" Over and over.

"Absolutely!" I answered again and again. "Of course I will." The problem was, I had no idea what that really meant. I had no idea how to hold people accountable.

Once I was in the job, I knew it was going to be a really bad day when a line of employees was outside my office door, waiting for me to arrive so they could complain about their coworkers.

"Can I talk with you about a problem?" I was asked ad nauseam. It got to the point where I would try to sneak into my office so I could have just a few minutes to get myself settled before getting hit with the avalanche of complaints. It was as though each morning they appointed a scout to watch for me at the entrance to the unit and sound the alarm, "She's here! She's here!" Well, at least it felt like that.

My employees would share things that shocked me. Like the time one of my night nurses walked off the unit even though the charge nurse told her that her patient just went into SVT. She walked off and said, "He's going to have to wait until I get back from my cigarette break." Or the time one of my patients coded, the LPN asked for help from one of my RNs but the RN walked right past her and said, "That's not my patient," and kept walking down the hallway.

Quality of care was a major issue. However, their behavior toward each other was even more disturbing. For example:

When my RN and LPN got into an argument at the nurses' station, the RN said, "You're not a real f****** nurse anyway!"

My unit secretary consistently hung up the phone on anyone she didn't want to talk to, marked her territory by yelling at anyone who touched "her" stapler, phone, or chair, and dropped the f-bomb when she got mad (which was frequently).

At least twice a week, I got called out to the nurses' station because someone refused to work with someone else. I received complaints from people outside of my department too. The way my employees treated pharmacy, radiology, other supervisors, support staff, etc. was embarrassing.

It got to the point that I would feel sick to my stomach as soon as I walked onto my unit and saw that line of people waiting for me.

How did I handle these complaints, accusations, and disturbing behaviors?

I did try to investigate, but every time, I would find out that there was another entirely different version of the story. Or, my employees would retaliate against me and call off if I confronted them. Other times, I was so overwhelmed that I just put the incident on the back burner with a plan to address it the next day. But the next day just delivered more problems. Many of the complaints never got addressed.

I questioned myself every day, and although I had good intent, I didn't know how to handle the numerous complaints. Sometimes, I took the wait-and-see approach.

If you're a leader reading this, I bet you've also put some of your employees' behaviors on the back burner too. If so, please don't beat yourself up as I did for over a decade after I quit that job!

It's time for a new approach! Building a culture that rejects any incidents of bullying and incivility happens when you stop using silence as a strategy and start addressing incidents of disruptive behaviors consistently over time.

In this chapter, we'll explore the following:

- How to confront disruptive behaviors using simple techniques

- How to create a process for addressing incidents of bad behavior with your employees

- How to document in a way that increases the likelihood that if you need to go down the disciplinary path, you'll be supported

Out of all of the content in this book, this chapter provides you with strategies and tactics that leaders like you tell me have made the biggest difference in transforming the culture in their department. This chapter is designed to help you switch from using silence as a strategy to actually confronting disruptive behaviors.

TECHNIQUES TO CONFRONT DISRUPTIVE BEHAVIORS

A primary reason leaders don't confront known or suspected bullying or uncivil behavior is that we don't know what to say or how to say it. What's more, it's extremely uncomfortable and stressful to confront someone about negative behavior. Many of us avoid confrontation at all costs. We justify why we don't speak up by minimizing the incidents (well, she's probably exaggerating), justifying (well, he's going through a divorce and I feel bad for him), or overlooking bad behavior because the employee is so competent (but she's a really great nurse!).

Sometimes leaders are afraid of confronting because they are concerned the employee will retaliate against them or the person who spoke up. Other times we get caught in the he said/she said trap, never knowing what the truth is, so we avoid confronting. "What if I'm wrong?" we ask ourselves.

Let's explore some simple confronting techniques that can provide you with a framework for addressing almost every type of behavior, even covert actions and behavior that you don't actually witness.

You may be skeptical and find yourself thinking that confronting doesn't work, so why should you bother to invest energy in learning these tactics. If so, your skepticism makes sense. The tactics I am about to share with you work—but not all of the time. Human behavior is complex. There is no one-size-fits-all when it comes to addressing someone's behavior. Not everyone is capable of adapting his or her behavior no matter how skillfully we confront it. Some disruptive employees need professional help. Let's acknowledge that confronting doesn't always work. *But not confronting never works!* We've been not confronting for decades. It's time to adopt a new strategy.

To get you started on the most productive path to successfully confronting disruptive behaviors, I'll teach you three powerful confronting techniques:

1. Name it

2. Speak it

3. Script it

Technique 1: Name It

Imagine Marie, one of my nurses, barging into my office and saying, "I can't stand working with Regina. She's such a bully!"

As a leader, what am I supposed to do with that information? I start with, "What did she do?"

Maria replies, "Regina is so condescending. She makes me feel like I'm stupid."

Again, what am I supposed to do with that? So I ask, "What did Regina say? What did she do to make you feel that way?"

To which Marie replies, "As soon as she saw that I was in charge, Regina threw her clipboard on the counter and said, in front of everyone, "Great! Today's going to be an awful day because you suck at being in charge!"

Now that is information I can do something about!

Bullying and incivility rarely end without intervention. Reducing disruptive behaviors requires confronting someone in a way that clearly and specifically identifies the inappropriate behavior, yet does so in a professional manner.

The simplest, easiest way to confront bullying or incivility is to *name the behavior.*

Naming the behavior as it occurs can stop things immediately and prevent an escalation of that behavior. Naming the behavior requires you and your employees to identify the behavior objectively because some nurses may not realize that their behavior is disruptive. When disruptive behavior is "named," it can help the perpetrator see himself or herself through the eyes of others.

Returning to our example, Regina threw her clipboard and yelled, "You suck at being in charge." When you name the behavior by saying, "You threw your clipboard and yelled, 'You suck at being in charge' in front of others..." you're now addressing a behavior—not labeling a person.

The key is to get very clear about the behavior someone is displaying that you believe is inappropriate. Then name it.

Here are some examples of "naming it":

- *You are **yelling and screaming** in the middle of the nurses' station where patients and families can hear you.*
- *You're **yelling** and need to stop right now.*
- *You just **threw** your clipboard.*
- *You're **huffing and puffing**.*

- *You just **dropped the f-bomb** in the hallway, in front of patients' rooms.*

Employees who feel a sense of power while yelling or throwing things gain momentum as they continue to act out; the longer they act out, the stronger the momentum. Typically, nobody says anything. Witnesses or those being yelled at may even turn or walk away, leaving the yeller to continue yelling. The simple act of naming the behavior (yelling and screaming, criticizing, etc.) can act like a defibrillator, stopping the yeller in his or her tracks.

Even eye rolling and mocking behavior can be named.

- *I just saw you **roll your eyes** when I asked you to help with a patient.*
- *I just heard you **mocking** him.*

Naming the behavior can send a message that you are not going to accept treating others in an unprofessional manner.

Several years ago, I held an adjunct faculty role at a local community college. One evening before class started, I was talking with a student when Jamie, another student, interrupted, "Dr. Thompson, where do I put this crap?" referring to her paperwork. At first, I didn't say anything because I was speaking to the other student.

Jamie repeated, "Dr. Thompson, where do I put this crap?"

I then stopped talking, looked at Jamie and said, "You put your paperwork here (pointing to the desk) and I want to see you after class."

Jamie replied, "Okay," and walked away as if nothing was wrong.

Jamie and I sat down after class, and I said, "Jamie, when you refer to your paperwork as *crap*, you are disrespecting me, your peers, and your school. I never want to hear you refer to anything as crap again. Okay? It's unprofessional and disrespectful."

As I named her behavior, Jamie's facial expressions went from cheery to melancholy. "Yes, Dr. Thompson," she said, and walked away.

I was curious about Jamie and asked one of the full-time instructors if she thought Jamie was a good student and would make a good nurse. As adjunct faculty, I didn't always have information about the students' behaviors or performance before or after their time with me. She said that Jamie had excellent clinical skills and would make a good nurse if she could control her potty mouth. She then gave me examples of other times when Jamie said inappropriate things in class. When I asked if anyone addressed Jamie's language, she said, "No. That's just Jamie, and if her future boss has a problem with her, she can address it."

We need to do better! We need to name behaviors we believe are unprofessional, disrespectful, and inappropriate. It's unprofessional of us to pass the behavior along to the next authority figure to deal with.

It's one thing to confront disruptive behavior when you witness it. What if you actually don't witness the behavior? Can you still name it? The answer is "yes."

For example, what if you have a nurse who reportedly throws a fit every time she gets an admission? It's to the point that the charge nurses just appease this nurse by doing everything they can to avoid giving her any admissions. This, of course, puts more of a burden on the other nurses, who are also sick of it. Multiple employees have complained, but of course, the nurse never behaves this way when you're around.

The first question to ask yourself is this: Do you believe the complaints are valid? If so, name the behavior. Speak to the nurse as follows, "It's been brought to my attention numerous times that you huff and puff, yell, and throw your clipboard on the counter when you're given an admission." The key here is to ask your staff to be very specific when they complain about her behavior. This way, your perpetrator will know you are serious, have investigated, and will not tolerate specific behaviors.

For example, it's better to say, "huff, puff, and throw your clipboard," than, "act unprofessionally." The more specific you can be, the better.

If you haven't done a good job addressing disruptive behavior in the past, start with naming it. It's the simplest and least emotionally uncomfortable tactic to confront disruptive behavior.

Randy, a nurse manager in an ICU, had an honest conversation with a patient care technician (PCT). When she saw her assignment at the beginning of a shift, this PCT made loud comments out at the nurses' station, expressing her frustrations with the assignment. During this conversation, Randy named her inappropriate behavior and coached her on methods she could have used. Together they set healthy workforce expectations and the next level consequence. There were tears, apologies, and hugs as she left smiling.

When it comes to unprofessional behavior in the workplace, it's not important that you understand why a person behaves a certain way, although that can be helpful. Focus on behaviors—let the psychologists focus on the reasons.

Technique 2: Speak It

Sixteen years ago, when I decided to step down from my role as a unit manager, I transferred into a clinician role on a neurosurgical unit managed by a very dear friend. Although they say you should never work for your friend, I felt I needed to be in an environment where I knew somebody cared about me.

After working on the unit for a few months, my friend (boss) called me into her office and said, "When my employees complain to me about one of their coworkers, I ignore them. When I hear the same complaint a second time, I pay attention. If I hear it a third time, I have a conversation with that employee."

As she was saying this, I was listening intently. After all, this was good stuff! Then she said, "Renee, I need to have a conversation with you."

"Me?" I answered, in shock. "Me? What have I done?"

She then told me that over the past month or so, several nurses had complained to her that when I worked night shift, I wasn't taking my patients down to radiology for their AM CT Scan.

"Yeah," I said. "It's an AM CT. That's the dayshift nurses' responsibility."

"No." she said. "It's the night nurses' responsibility to take all patients ordered a CT in AM down before they leave their shift."

At first I was mortified that I had been so careless and failed to complete my work, causing more work for the dayshift nurses. However, after I got over my initial shock and embarrassment, I got angry and said, "Do you mean to tell me that these nurses complained to you about this but never had the courtesy of being honest with me?" Basically, when I would give report, they wouldn't say anything to me, but as soon as I left for home, they went running to the boss to tattle on me. Contrast this with another situation in which I unknowingly made a mistake.

I was new to the med/surg observation unit. At the time, I had been a nurse for 24 years but hadn't practiced at the bedside for a while. A lot of things had changed since I was at the bedside, but I was bound and determined to catch up.

One weekend, Mike, a night nurse, took over my assignment. I was scheduled to work the following morning and took assignment back from Mike. After bedside report, Mike said to me, "Oh, by the way, you didn't complete the admission patient education documentation on the patient you admitted yesterday."

I replied, "Tony did the actual admission for me."

Mike replied, "It's not Tony's responsibility to do the patient education documentation. It's yours."

I had been working on the unit for a few months and had never thought to check the admission paperwork after the admission nurse admitted the patient! I assumed that he or she completed everything related to the admission.

I said to Mike, "Let me get this straight—even if someone else admits a patient for me, I need to go back into the education documentation to make sure everything was completed?"

"Absolutely," he said. "Let me show you." And then he showed me his method for checking to make sure everything was done.

What's the difference between the first and second situation?

In the first situation, none of my coworkers gave me the courtesy of being honest with me. Instead, they were dishonest and disrespectful by going behind my back.

In the second situation, Mike showed me respect by being honest with me. Mike didn't judge and didn't assume. He just informed.

Mike was willing to *speak it.*

Effective, respectful, and professional communication is a foundation of a healthy workforce culture and the ability to deliver high-quality and safe patient care. We can all improve workplace communication by striving to be as proficient in communication skills as we are in clinical skills.

Of course, you and your employees are not all skilled in effective communication, are you? Here's why: All humans communicate using one of four primary communication styles: aggressive, passive, passive-aggressive, and assertive. When it comes to being honest and respectful, you'll find that each of the four styles lands in a different place.

Before we can learn to speak it, we have to do a quick review of the four communication styles.

Aggressive style communicators are honest with you, but they are not very respectful. In fact, people who use this style are exceedingly blunt. People who communicate using the aggressive style may even get right in your face, yell, scream, and openly criticize others. They have a need to be right and may not easily see situations from the perspective of others. These employees tend to be the ones who don't wait in line to complain to you about their coworkers—they handle situations on their own! On the flip side, aggressive employees are frequently the ones other employees complain about.

Passive style communicators aren't honest, but it's because they are so intent on being respectful. They won't tell you the truth because they don't want to hurt your feelings or they are afraid of how you will respond. People who use this style are exceedingly considerate for fear of conflict or stepping on toes, however, they are not always honest about their true feelings. People-pleasers often fall in this category. They may never complain to you, but may be really struggling with their coworkers.

Passive-aggressive style communicators are neither nice nor respectful. These are the people who act nice, even sweet, to your face, but as soon as you turn around, they are stabbing you in the back. When asked directly why they are angry or upset, they may act bitter, chilly, or stoic, or they may smile and say nothing is wrong, yet continue to give you the cold shoulder. These are the employees who tattle on each other, spread rumors, gossip, and complain, but fail to provide the entire story. Of all the types of communicators on a team, passive-aggressive communicators are the most exhausting ones to deal with. As an example, my colleagues on the neuro unit communicated using the passive-aggressive communication style. They said nothing to me (passive) but then tattled to our boss (aggressive).

Assertive style communicators strive to be honest and respectful at the same time. This is a direct, strong, and calm style of communication which focuses on achieving healthy compromises that respect everyone involved. This style, without contest, is the most effective for healthcare as well as most other environments. Mike utilized the assertive communication style—he was honest (you didn't do the paperwork) and respectful (I'll show you how).

Unfortunately, the assertive communication style is least used in healthcare.

Most of us communicate in the style we learned from our first family and have adapted to match our personalities. If we deal with frustration by yelling, chances are we had a parent who modeled that for us. If we give people the silent treatment when we are hurt or offended, chances are someone did the same to us when we were children. And, to some extent, the way we communicate on our units reflects the style modeled for us when we first began in healthcare.

The good news is that once we begin to observe the behaviors of our own communication style, we can adjust those behaviors to be healthier and more effective. In other words, we can learn the assertive communication style, even if it doesn't come naturally to us. Assertive communication is a skill. Here are some of the observable behaviors of an assertive communicator:

- Articulates concerns directly to the person with whom he or she has an issue; avoids talking about someone behind his or her back

- Listens actively and reflectively to others

- Offers direct eye contact

- Maintains a relaxed posture when talking to others

- Communicates positively and constructively, without judging or labeling

- Uses words like "we" and "our"

- Focuses on the goal, not on self

- Encourages the other person to explain before jumping to conclusions

- Communicates with honesty and with respect

Your goal, as the leader, is to develop your assertive communication skills and help your employees do the same.

For a copy of the Develop Assertive Communication Skills Tip Sheet, visit the resource vault at https://theHealthyWorkforceInstitute.com/Resource-Vault

A nurse manager who had been working with her team on developing assertive communication skills shared the following:

> Recently a charge nurse pulled an employee aside to a private area and discussed an incident that had just happened. She immediately addressed the behavior and said, "Let's talk about what happened and how we might have been able to handle the situation differently."
>
> She did not wait or run to management, expecting us to address the staff member. As a charge nurse, she respectfully shared feedback and addressed the situation in real time. She shared with us what happened

following the incident so we could be aware and stay informed. It was a great example of effective leadership!

As the leader, you want to serve as a role model of assertive communication in all your conversations. As we discussed in Chapter 3, engaging in honest and respectful conversations with your employees about their behavior is essential to transforming the culture in your department. Although it may be uncomfortable to be direct and honest with your employees, especially if you're concerned about how they will respond, developing your assertive communication skills is a must if you are ever going to create a healthy workforce culture!

However, don't expect to magically start communicating assertively overnight. It takes time and practice to adapt your communication style, especially if you've established a strong preference for a different style. Start small but start *now*. Here is a good beginning practice:

The Power of the Pause

I've talked with many, many leaders who have caught themselves being reactive in the moment when dealing with employees who misbehave. For example, one leader, Yvonne, shared that her organization launched a new process for getting IV pumps. Instead of hoarding pumps in their supply room, as the nurses often did, pumps would need to be ordered from the central supply department for a specific patient. When that patient no longer needed the IV pump, the pump would have to be sent back to the central supply department.

One of Yvonne's older, experienced night nurses, Helen, was outraged and complained about the new policy to

Yvonne and anyone else who would listen. One day, Yvonne walked onto the unit in the morning and saw a large red sign on their supply room that said, "New stupid process for IV pumps that wastes our time. Ask Yvonne."

Yvonne was furious. She immediately ripped down the sign, stormed into the nurses' station where Helen was sitting and yelled, "I know this was you, Helen! How would you like it if I posted signs on your locker about everything I don't like about you?" Everyone stopped what he or she was doing and watched Yvonne, their leader, behave in a way that was aggressive, unprofessional, and inappropriate.

When Yvonne shared this experience with me, she knew she had reacted harshly, and she asked for advice on how she should have responded. I suggested that anytime she feels herself getting angry about a situation at work, to first pause, take a deep breath, and say to herself, "How can I handle this situation with honesty and respect?" The way Yvonne had reacted to Helen was unprofessional in at least two ways:

First, she assumed Helen posted that sign, which may or may not have turned out to be accurate. She could have said, "Yvonne. Did you post this sign on the supply room door? It looks like your handwriting."

Second, once she confirmed that Helen had posted the sign, she could have taken Helen into her office to discuss the inappropriateness of her actions. Doing this prevents distracting everyone else from their work by causing a scene at the nurses' station.

When speaking with any nurse about disruptive behavior, I suggested that Yvonne name the behavior (posting sign on door), identify the impact (undermines her authority; patients and families can see this which may cause them anxiety, etc.), and reinforce that the behavior was unprofessional, disrespectful, and inappropriate.

This incident was Yvonne's opportunity as the leader to show Helen what respect and professionalism look like. She might have said to Helen, "I want to talk to you about how you handled this situation. I understand you were up-set about the changes, but as a professional nurse and as someone who has worked here for a very long time, I ex-pect you to model professionalism even when you disa-gree. The way you handled this situation was not okay. Can we talk about how you could have handled this different-ly?"

Now, in full disclosure, Helen's behavior was extremely inappropriate and did lead to disciplinary action, as it should have. But Yvonne missed the opportunity to set a positive example and tone for how employees handle diffi-cult situations. Employees model their behavior on the ex-amples and expectations that their leaders set.

Before you engage in a conversation with one of your employees, pause, take a deep breath, and think: How can I be honest and respectful at the same time? How can I serve as a role model of professional communication? How can I stop myself from being reactive?

It starts with a good pause before speaking.

Technique 3: Script It

"That's not my job," said Matt, one of the nursing assistants on Debbie's unit. During the staff meeting, Debbie, the unit manager, had just informed her employees that in an at-tempt to improve their patient satisfaction scores, they were asking everyone to keep an eye on the cleanliness of their rooms. If they saw overfilled trash cans, a dirty floor, or excessive clutter, they were to clean it up.

Debbie froze. She felt herself get flustered and didn't know what to say. She chose to ignore Matt and continue the meeting. For the rest of the day, however, she couldn't help thinking about how rude Matt was and about how ineffectively she had handled it. Debbie mentally beat herself up for not addressing his behavior as she replayed the scene over and over in her mind like a bad movie.

Has this ever happened to you? Have you ever been in a situation where someone embarrassed you or undermined your authority in front of others? Have you ever actually seen or heard one of your employees openly criticize another employee or display strong offensive body language while talking to support staff? What about finding out that your employee flipped out at the nurses' station because he didn't like his assignment?

When these situations happen, I'm guessing you are a lot like me: You get caught off guard and can't think of what to say or what to do in the moment. But the next day in the shower, oh! You can think of all sorts of things to say! But by then, it's too late.

A powerful tactic for addressing someone's disruptive behavior in the moment is to prepare ahead of time with a script. A script is the main group of words that supports the rest of the conversation. Like the stem on a tree that supports the smaller branches, identifying an appropriate script, followed by specifics, supports your ability to address common disruptive behaviors.

Here are some of my favorites:

- *Help me to understand ...*
- *I'm not sure you're aware ...*
- *I'm concerned about ...*
- *I'm offended by that comment ...*
- *I've noticed that ...*

When you witness someone being disruptive (yelling, cursing, etc.), as a leader, it's important that you immediately stop the behavior by naming it, which is basically using a script, such as:

- *You are yelling ... and need to stop.*
- *I just heard you say the f-word.*
- *What you just said is offensive.*

But what if you don't actually witness someone's bad behavior but you know you need to address it?

Scripting works well in these situations too!

Start with a powerful script, and then add the specific situation or behavior (name it). Here are some examples:

Script:
Help Me to Understand ...

- *...why you are assigning the newest nurses the toughest assignments (and then provide specifics).*
- *It was brought to my attention that _____ occurred. Help me to understand what happened.*

Stating "help me to understand," decreases defensiveness, just a bit. The employee is more likely to engage in a conversation about the situation rather than argue with you. As we all know, sometimes there is more to a story than what we originally thought.

Script:
I'm concerned about ...

- *... the way you handled the situation yesterday. I'm not sure you realize how your behavior affected ... (patient satisfaction, the way our team communicates with each other, quality care, etc.).*

- *... the way you behave when asked to take an admission (then give a specific example).*

- *... how you treat new employees here (then provide specific behaviors).*

Script:
I'm not sure you're aware ...

or

I'm not sure you realize ...

- *... that sometimes you come across as being unapproachable ... (give specifics)*

- *... that sometimes you communicate aggressively ... (give specifics)*

- *... that sometimes you get very reactive ... (give specifics)*

Note: Any time you use the script, "I'm not sure you're aware," back it up with a recent example.

- *Just yesterday (or this morning) I saw how you reacted when Tracy told you that you were getting an admission. You huffed, sighed, and then stomped away from the nurses' station murmuring to yourself. You didn't notice that Tracy got upset. There was also a family member standing at the nurses' station who saw how you reacted.*

Many leaders don't think they can counsel an employee about disruptive behavior if they don't exactly witness it. This is where scripting can be really helpful!

Melinda, a secretary on a unit, was in the habit of cursing like a truck driver right in the nurses' station. Of course, she never behaved that way when the manager, Luke, was around. Luke didn't think he could confront Melinda because he had never heard her curse. I asked Luke if he believed Melinda cursed at the nurses' station, he replied, "Absolutely."

If you believe it to be true and you've determined that this is a pattern of disruptive behavior, you must counsel this employee using scripting techniques. I told Luke to schedule a meeting with Melinda, sit face-to-face (same level), and then use the following script:

Script:
It's been brought to my attention that ...

- *... you've been cursing at the nurses' station where patients and their families can hear you (it's always good to include patients whenever you can). Although I've never heard you curse, I believe this is true.*

Note: Your employee might get very defensive and say, "Who said something? Who complained?" This is an attempt to distract you. Don't let this happen! Say this, "It doesn't matter who told me. I believe that you are cursing and we need to talk about it."

- *It is my expectation, and the expectation of this organization and our department (you can refer back to your department norms) that we refrain from any profanity, yelling, or disrespectful language, especially in patient care areas. Cursing is a never event.*

- *Starting in this moment, I never want to find out that you've cursed at the nurses' station or anywhere a patient or family member can hear you.*

Let's revisit the incident in which Matt made rude comments while Debbie, his manager, was asking all staff members to pull together to keep the entire unit clean. What could Debbie have done to address Matt's rude comments during the staff meeting?

It's the same scripted response for employees like Matt, who say, "That's not my job," or any other rude, inconsiderate, or disrespectful comments that reflect a lack of commitment for the work.

Say this:

- *When you say _____ (I don't care, that's not my job, etc.), in healthcare, that concerns me (script).*

- *We are all asked to do things that are beyond our job description for the sake of somebody's mother, father, spouse, etc.*

- *If you "don't care" or aren't willing to do things beyond your job description, perhaps this job isn't a good fit for you.*

Don't let your employees get away with rude or disrespectful comments. Address them immediately. In healthcare, when everything we do or don't do impacts someone's life, we're all asked to go above and beyond our job description—we're all asked to care.

For more scripting examples visit the Heathy Workforce Institute Resource Vault at
https://theHealthyWorkforceInstitute.com/Resource-Vault

Disruptive behaviors happen because they can. It takes willing individuals and leaders to stop it. Of course, becoming proficient at naming it, speaking it, and scripting it won't happen overnight. All skills take practice. But each time you confront disruptive behavior clearly and directly, you make a small change in the culture of your unit or department.

Chad Green, PACU manager, shared the results of his journey to confronting misbehavior in the following way:

> I have fewer complaints, and although they still happen, I address them more quickly and with less dread than I did before. Depending on what the complaint is, I may talk to the individual privately, but many times the complaint is something that can be addressed with the entire staff. One big difference is that I am better at having these conversations than I was before. I also challenge any staff bringing a complaint to have a conversation with the other person, and then I follow up to see if that conversation has taken place.

Follow Chad's lead by trying the techniques in this chapter. You'll be amazed at how quickly this changes your confidence as a leader as well as the behavior of your staff.

Of all of the strategies to eradicate bullying and incivility, confronting is usually met with the most trepidation. Think about it. Many leaders have used silence as a strategy because they try to avoid conflict at all costs! However, now that you're equipped with a few powerful confronting techniques, confronting doesn't have to feel as painful as you once thought. The best way to go from silence to confronting is to start small. Just choose a few scripts you can use in the moment; a few common behaviors that you can "name"; and a few tactics to speak using the assertive communication style (honest and respectful). The key is to start! Like the late great Martin Luther King, Jr. said, "Take the first step in faith. You don't have to see the whole staircase, just the first step."

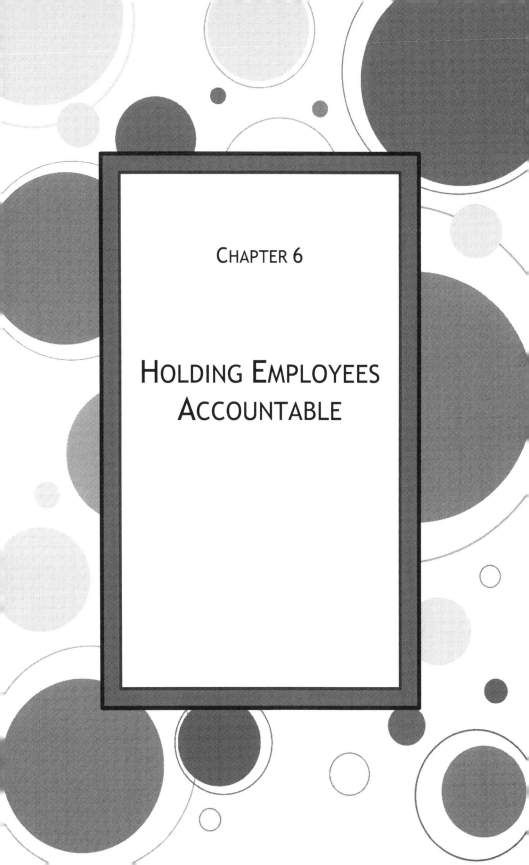

CHAPTER 6

HOLDING EMPLOYEES ACCOUNTABLE

The key to success is to get the right people on the bus and get the wrong people off the bus. Then, put the right people in the right seats on the bus.

~Jim Collins

CHAPTER 6

HOLDING EMPLOYEES ACCOUNTABLE

Kayla, the manager on the med/surg oncology unit, had been dealing with high turnover and poor retention because of a single toxic person. This person, otherwise known as "The Beast," had been wreaking havoc on the unit for decades. His toxic behavior had never been addressed because he was so clinically competent. Finally, Kayla had enough and decided to terminate The Beast. When she contacted HR, however, she hit a brick wall. The HR representative asked the following questions:

- What have you done to help him change his behavior?

- Have you crossed all of your *t's* and dotted your *i's*?

- Well, did you counsel him? How many times have you counseled him? Only five? Oh, you need to at least counsel him 27 times before we can take any action (I'm exaggerating a bit).

- And on and on ...

Unfortunately, this story repeats itself daily. When front line managers finally decide to do something about their problem employees, they don't always get the support they need or expect from HR. Managers complain all the time about how HR never supports them, especially if a union represents their employees. Lack of support from HR is probably one of the top five complaints I hear from managers.

But is HR really the brick wall you think they are?

You might be surprised to learn that when a healthcare organization reaches out to me for help, at least 40% of the inbound requests come from someone in HR. This means they're aware of the problem and don't necessarily have the solution either. Spending time with folks in HR has afforded me the opportunity to see the world through their eyes.

For example, Sanja, an HR business partner for the inpatient nursing units in a hospital, received a call from Gary, the manager of a medical ICU. Gary insisted that Sanja meet with him that day because he had an urgent need. When Gary entered Sanja's office, he was outwardly upset, refused to sit down, and said, "You need to approve a termination! I've had enough with her behavior. That's it. I'm done!"

Apparently, Gary had been dealing with a toxic employee, Rita, who had never been held accountable for her behavior. He had just lost another new nurse because of Rita. Gary had been the manager on that unit for more than 10 years and had witnessed Rita's covert, pot-stirring, sneaky, sabotaging methods to squash anyone she didn't like for all that time. Gary had had enough. He didn't care how great Rita was clinically.

After listening to Gary rant and rave about Rita, Sanja found herself unable to approve the termination, leaving Gary outraged. Brick wall? Not so fast. Here's why:

In the 10+ years Gary had been dealing with Rita's be-havior, he had never mentioned her name to Sanja, his HR business partner. He had no real documentation about Rita's behavior, just an anecdotal paragraph written on a notepad.

When Sonya looked back at Rita's performance reviews for the last 15 years, the records showed she had received "meets" or "exceeds expectations" on every single review. How was Sanja supposed to justify a termination when there was no shred of documentation that Rita was disrup-tive?

This story represents a disconnect between a front line leader and his HR partners, a condition widespread in healthcare.

Many front line managers view HR as the last resort to get the help they need to discipline or terminate an em-ployee for disruptive behavior. HR, however, can't help if the manager hasn't built a case that warrants corrective action.

I know because I also experienced the disconnect I'm talking about. When I was a unit manager and realized how toxic some of my employees were, I decided to take action. Unfortunately, I discovered that nothing had been documented in their employee files by the previous man-agers, so when I came to HR for help, I got the run around. I was told repeatedly that I didn't have enough "ammuni-tion" and, therefore, couldn't take any action. It took me over a year to terminate three of my toxic employees! But by then, I had lost some really great employees who just couldn't tolerate working in that environment.

Almost every time I host a workshop for leaders on the topic of bullying, a manager will approach me at the end and say, "That's it! I'm going to go back and *fire* my bully!" Whoa! Unfortunately, you can't fire someone just because today you decide that enough is enough.

In this chapter, we'll explore the following:

- How to create a process for addressing incidents of bad behavior with your employees

- How to document in a way that increases the likelihood you'll be supported by HR if you need to go down the disciplinary path

- How to use an effective interview process to hire the right people

- How to effectively confront a nurse who is clinically competent but toxic to those around him or her

CREATE A PROCESS FOR ADDRESSING INCIDENTS OF BAD BEHAVIOR

Leaders have the responsibility to listen and take action when receiving complaints of any behavior that violates policy, patient care, or team performance. However, as we've discussed, many leaders use avoidance or silence as a strategy because they don't know how to handle the situation and/or they don't feel supported by their HR department.

Organizations typically have a clearly defined disciplinary or corrective action process—verbal warning, written warning, suspension, and eventually termination—when it comes to objective, tangible violations like time and attendance issues. Oh, it's easy to hold someone accountable who calls off 57 times! However, I've not yet seen an organization that has a clearly defined process for how to handle *initial* complaints of bullying or incivility.

For example, what do you do when you start getting complaints that the experienced nurse you just hired is rude, condescending, and abrasive to the staff? Do you talk to her? Just start a documentation trail? Ignore it? What reference or resource would you use as a guide? Would you call your HR business partner right away or wait? I challenge you to find a process for these types of complaints in your policies!

If you can't find a process for how to handle complaints of disruptive behavior beyond your organization's disciplinary path, which we know doesn't necessarily address acts of bullying and incivility, it's time to adopt one.

Of course, you typically won't witness someone's initial disruptive behavior yourself, but you'll find out about it through a series of employee complaints. As the leader, you are still responsible for addressing the behavior and starting a process to eliminate it.

It distresses me that many employees tell me that when they complain to their manager about someone's behavior, they often get told just to ignore the person, to stop being so sensitive, or that it's just their personality and not to take them seriously.

When an employee complains about his or her coworker's behavior, it's your job to take that complaint seriously. Please don't say, "You're being too sensitive; I'm sure he didn't mean anything by it;" or "That's just her personality." Instead say, "I believe you. Now let's talk about this."

Ask questions in a way that helps you determine if this was a one-time incident (having a bad day) or if this behavior is more serious. Did this person's behavior impact patients in any way? Has this employee behaved this way before? Sometimes, by the time an employee complains about a coworker, the complainant has been dealing with the behavior for a while.

If this is the first time you're hearing about someone's disruptive behavior, start paying attention. Look for any evidence that this employee might be treating others the same way. Do similar complaints from others come to mind? Develop a heightened sense of awareness about this employee to discover if the complaints about his or her disruptive behavior are valid and indicate a pattern. Once you decide that the complaints are valid, it's time to follow a formal process.

Anytime you personally witness disruptive behavior (yelling, openly criticizing, etc.) it's your responsibility to stop the behavior immediately using the "name it" technique we discussed in Chapter 5. But what do you do after stopping the behavior? Do you just go back to what you were working on? Let your employee go back to what he or she was working on?

That's what we might want to do. Stopping someone's disruptive behavior in the moment is a great first step; however, if you want to create and sustain a professional workforce culture, you have to take the next step. You have to schedule time with the disruptive employee to discuss the behavior.

Once you and the employee have calmed down, ask to speak with him or her in your office or other private location. And then have an informal conversation.

First Incident: Informal Conversation

The goal is to engage in a collegial conversation with your employee about the behavior you witnessed or have validated. Just like having a conversation with someone over a cup of coffee, you're simply having a conversation. Start by saying, "I want to talk with you about what happened this morning (afternoon, yesterday, etc.)." Then follow this process:

Name the Behavior
I saw how you reacted when Nancy told you that you were getting an admission. You huffed, threw your hands in the air, and walked away, stomping down the hallway, complaining.

Add Impact
You behaved this way in the hallway, in front of patients' rooms where they and their family members could hear you. Not only could your behavior impact patients and their families, but when you act unprofessionally in front of your peers, it creates stress and anxiety among the team. It's not okay to behave that way.

Be Respectful
Can we talk about this? What happened?

Give the employee an opportunity to explain his or her side of the story. Listen with compassion. This person may be going through a difficult time. However, as we've discussed before, bad behavior is never justified, just sometimes understood.

Reinforce Expectations

As employees on this unit and professional nurses, we all agreed to _____ (this is where you would refer to the specific expectations in your department norms). I never want to see you behave that way again or find out from someone else that you acted so unprofessionally. Can I count on you not to behave that way again?

Document Your Conversation

Even though this is an informal conversation, it's important that you document what you witnessed and the conversation you had with your employee. Don't use your brain as a file cabinet! Document the conversation. We'll explore how best to document shortly.

Finally, let your employee know that the conversation you just had isn't official counseling. Explain that you want to give the employee an opportunity to step up as a professional and that the incident won't be included in his or her official employee file. In doing this, you are indicating that you believe the employee can do better and that you're willing to give him or her the opportunity to do so.

Note: You have a 72-hour window to engage in a conversation with your employee about his or her behavior once an incident occurs. Studies show that if you're going to give someone feedback about behavior, it's best to give that feedback within 72 hours. Any longer than that, the employee will forget the details and so will you!

Second Incident: Formal Conversation

If the behavior happens again, it's time to have a formal conversation. Schedule a private meeting with your employee for this conversation, and follow this process:

Name the Behavior Again

It was brought to my attention ... or ... I observed how you acted when you got an admission. Be specific. *This is the second time we're having a conversation about your disruptive behavior.*

Remind Them of Your Agreement

When we met the last time (include date), you said I could count on you to be respectful when getting an admission. What happened? You did not honor our agreement.

Using the word "honor" triggers an emotional response; it shows that you're disappointed.

Counsel

You might want to ask the employee what she can do to manage emotions when faced with admissions he or she doesn't like. You might offer her suggestions and encourage the employee to get support from other resources, such as friends and family, or EAP, especially when struggling with personal issues. Use this opportunity to support and counsel your employee. This is your job as the leader. However, make it very clear although you may empathize, any incidents of disruptive behaviors will not be tolerated.

Identify Consequences If the Behavior Continues

I'm documenting this incident as official counseling and citing this conversation as a verbal warning in your employee file. I still believe you can do better. If I witness or find out that you've behaved this way again,

I'll create an action plan for you to adhere to and schedule biweekly meetings with you to make sure you're following the plan. If you violate the action plan, you could be terminated.

Reinforce Expectations
I expect you to adhere to our department norms.

At this point, contact your HR business partner and let your representative know about this employee, his or her behavior, and what you've done so far. Don't wait until you're at your wit's end before you give HR a heads up!

Recently, I was coaching two nurse leaders who needed my help with their charge nurse. The charge nurse had been on the unit for decades, was clinically competent, and was the clique leader among a very strong group of employees. The situation had gotten so bad that the employees truly viewed the charge nurse as having more power than the managers. They shared numerous examples of how disruptive she was, from demonstrating simple favoritism to engaging in covert sabotage.

These managers, who were enrolled in my course, *Eradicating Bullying & Incivility*, finally made the decision to start this charge nurse down the disciplinary path. When we met, they had just had another significant incident with her and were trying to decide whether to give her a final written warning or just terminate her.

My first question was, "Did you give your HR business partner a heads up?" It was obvious by the looks on their faces that they had not.

I said, "As soon as our session is over, immediately call your HR business partner and tell her exactly what you just told me."

When leaders keep their HR representative in the loop, they are more likely to get their support when and if they decide to terminate an employee.

Third Incident: Corrective Action

Once you reach this step, carefully follow your organization's formal disciplinary process.

When dealing with disruptive behavior, start with an informal conversation and then formalize the process if the behavior continues. Give your HR representative, and perhaps your boss, a head's up on what's been happening. Once you identify an employee who might be heading down the disciplinary path for disruptive behavior, keep both in the loop.

Michelle, a director on a med/surg unit, followed the steps in this chapter to change the culture in her unit. Michelle, like many front line leaders, struggled with confronting employees and holding them accountable for their behavior. Michelle often got caught in the he said/she said battle, was reluctant to confront someone until she had conducted a thorough investigation (which was always sidelined for more pressing issues), and was inconsistent regarding documentation and corrective action. Morale was low, turnover was high, and Michelle questioned whether or not she had what it takes to be a leader.

One of her nurses, Judy, had been a problem from the beginning. If Judy didn't like her assignment, she would change it. Judy was known for making the new nurses cry, treating float staff terribly, and refusing to take report from any nurse she didn't deem worthy of her time. Although Michelle knew Judy's behavior was a problem, Michelle was a bit intimidated by her and, as a result, found every excuse for avoiding confrontation with her.

Michelle realized she had difficulties confronting any negative behavior on the unit and sought help. She learned how to "name it," "speak it," and "script it." She had some successes using the process outlined in this chapter for addressing incidents of disruptive behavior and began building a relationship with her HR business partner. Michelle began to feel more confident in her ability to lead her team. It was time to tackle Judy.

Michelle invited Judy to her office for a chat (informal conversation). During this chat, Michelle let Judy know that while she was clinically competent, she didn't behave in a professional manner (honest conversation). Michelle set the expectation for a healthy workforce and asked Judy to step up. Michelle let Judy know that she was counting on her, as an experienced and competent nurse, to be the role model for professionalism.

The very next day Judy got visibly angry when the charge nurse told her she was getting an admission. Judy stormed down the hallway and delayed the admission. When Michelle found out, she asked to meet with Judy privately.

Michelle reminded Judy of their conversation the previous day, asked what happened (I thought you said I could count on you ...), and then let Judy know that her behavior was unacceptable. She informed Judy that she was documenting their conversation as official counseling, which would become a part of Judy's permanent record. Michelle repeated her expectations.

A week later, Judy misbehaved again. This time, Michelle contacted Tammy, her HR business partner, to give her a heads up. Michelle and Tammy created a performance improvement plan and got approval from Michelle's boss. Michelle and Tammy presented the plan to Judy and informed Judy that they were to meet weekly to review her progress. Judy continued to misbehave, and three weeks later, Michelle and Tammy decided it was time to "therapeutically extract" Judy from the organization. Because Michelle had involved Tammy early on, all of the required documentation was complete and the termination was processed quickly.

For Michelle, going through the uncomfortable process of corrective action with an employee felt less stressful because she and Tammy went through the process together. She knew Tammy supported her!

Buoyed by her success, Michelle began to consistently set behavioral expectations, confront disruptive behaviors immediately, follow a consistent process, and involve an HR representative early on. It didn't take long before Michelle saw a dramatic change in her department. Morale improved and turnover dropped. Michelle had led a culture change by holding employees accountable. You can too!

* * * * *

Without documentation, it's impossible to hold employees accountable to the point of disciplinary action. To lead effectively, you must build the skill of documenting in a way that clearly articulates how an employee's behavior is negatively impacting patients, the team, or the organization.

First, get into the habit of documenting any conversations you have with your employees about behavioral expectations and any reports of bullying, incivility, or unprofessional behavior. You can do this in a variety of ways:

- Create an electronic document for each employee where you can add an entry.

- Use your organization's form (if one exists) for documenting conversations.

- Keep a running, written document on your computer that you can cut and paste into an employee's electronic file.

The choice of "how" is up to you; just pick a system for documentation—and use it consistently.

To find an example of a documentation template, go to https://theHealthyWorkforceInstitute.com/Resource-Vault.

WHAT TO INCLUDE IN YOUR DOCUMENTATION

Date and Time
Always, always, always include the date and time that you either witnessed disruptive behaviors or received a report about them. Without a date, your documentation is almost invalid.

Location
Note where the incident occurred. Be sure to state, "in the nurses' station; in room 4214; in the hallway on unit 5N, in classroom 2," etc.

Incident

Describe the incident as objectively as possible. Stick with the facts! Do not include your opinions. Leave out any justifications or reasons why this person behaved this way. Only document objective behaviors. This works even when an employee complains about someone else's behavior. Write down exactly what they say happened.

Witnesses

Include the names of anyone who was present when the incident occurred. This works best if you actually witnessed the behavior. Including witnesses, even if those witnesses are not willing to document, lends credibility to your documentation and helps with the investigative process.

Include Verbatim Comments

Make sure to include anything the employee actually said in your documentation. For example, when I shared the story about my nursing assistant who threatened my nurse, everyone documented that she said: "My boyfriend knows what shuttle you take and is going to be waiting for you to beat the s*** out of you!" It's very powerful when you can actually quote something someone says.

Use Language in Policy, Code of Conduct, and Department Norms

This is why it's so important for you to know your policies regarding professional conduct and that you've created department norms—you can now use the language from these policies and norms in your documentation. It's about helping your HR department clearly see how someone's behavior has violated expectations for professional conduct. Make it easy for your HR business partner and you'll have a better chance of getting that person's support.

Link Behavior to a Patient Safety, Quality, Satisfaction Concern, or Team Communication

If a behavior doesn't impact patients or the way the team communicates with each other, it might not be worth your time and energy. But when a behavior does have negative impact in any of these areas, you, as a leader, have an ethical responsibility to take action. In your documentation, link someone's behavior to patients or the team. To determine if an episode of unprofessional or disruptive behavior is worth documenting, ask yourself, "So what?"

- So what if someone rolled her eyes at you?

- So what if someone likes creamy peanut butter but you like chunky?

- So what if an experienced nurse refused to take report from the new nurse?

If after asking "So what?" you can clearly see how specific disruptive behavior impacts patients or the team, document it. If it doesn't, don't waste your time. Why? Because you are far less likely to get support to carry out any disciplinary action.

Let me be clear: Deciding not to document a behavior doesn't mean you can't have a conversation about it. But any documentation needs to be clear and focused on the behavior and negative impact to patients or the team.

Remember, when employees run into your office complaining about their coworkers and then refuse to document, you can still document the conversation. Just follow the steps above and document.

I know documentation takes time, energy, and sometimes a healthy dose of moral courage! But I'm telling you, if you want to create a healthy workforce and stop bad behavior, it's worth your time. In fact, it's essential.

Even if you go to HR for help and they do nothing, documentation shows proof that you asked for help; it creates a trail of evidence.

HWF BEST PRACTICE TIP

DOCUMENTATION

Anna, an associate CNO enrolled in my *Eradicating Bullying & Incivility* course, shared her approach to documentation. She said, "I document on my employees the way I documented on my patients when I worked bedside."

This is brilliant!

Think about it. Before the end of every shift as a nurse, you had to make sure you had documented your care. Documentation is the number one reason for overtime in healthcare! Nurses are so busy providing care for patients throughout their shifts that they don't always have time to document that care as it occurs. Many finish patient care, give report, and then sit down to document.

Front line managers need to do the same thing.

Before you leave for the day, document any incidents of disruptive behaviors, counseling, or "coffee" conversations you had with employees. Make it a habit.

Start documenting as soon as you sense a problem and begin a conversation with an employee about disruptive behavior. Frame it in a way that links disruptive behavior to organization goals.

Use an Effective Interview Process to Hire the Right People

Have you ever interviewed someone you thought was a perfect fit for your unit? Perhaps she was a nurse who had experience, was already certified and educated, dressed professionally, and was articulate and nice! Of course you hired her, patted yourself on the back, and hoped that you could find 10 more just like her! Then, two months later, you discovered this new nurse you had hired was the wicked witch. Now you regularly have employees in your office, sometimes crying, because of how she treats them. What went wrong?

Did this nurse suddenly develop a split personality? Are you in the movie *Body Snatchers*? No. More likely, you missed something during the interviewing process.

Bad hires are expensive and can cost an organization as much as $50,000. And we all know that one bad apple can spoil the barrel. Studies show that rudeness is contagious. Hire one rude, toxic employee and you are likely to see a domino effect; they all start to fall to that standard.

In my various roles of nurse manager years ago, I interviewed many nurses and nursing assistants. During one of our most profound nursing shortages, I was tempted to hire anyone who had an active license and breathed. However, I knew the importance of hiring the right person.

Interviewing is not one of my strongest skills. In fact, it's as easy to bamboozle me as nearly everyone else during an interview. We see the good in people and think everyone is so nice! I hired people I thought were amazing who turned out to be Attila the Hun reincarnated. Others who I didn't think would be a good fit turned out to be my best hires.

Knowing how so much depends upon hiring the right people, I finally got smart and learned an effective interviewing strategy.

Use Behavioral Interviewing Techniques

Behavioral interviewing allows you to assess how well someone has performed in the past so that you can assess if that person will fit in well within your organization. If you want to avoid hiring a bully, asking behavioral based questions is essential! Here are a few to choose from:

- *Tell me what kind of people you find difficult to work with.*

- *Give me an example of a conflict at work and how you handled it.*

- *Give me an example of when you've made a mistake and how you dealt with it.*

- *Describe a stressful situation and how you handled it.*

Use Group Interviews

Some people can totally ace these behavioral questions and still not be a good fit. These individuals know the right language, and they may have preplanned and rehearsed "right answers" to the most common behavioral questions. Your staff, not being trained in interviewing techniques, may catch interviewees off guard by asking questions they hadn't anticipated. Further, in asking your staff to interview the potential hire, you're tapping into the collective power of others who might ultimately be better than you at interviewing. As a bonus, they feel more involved in the process and will make sure this person is a good fit! The stakes for your staff members are high, and they know it.

Ask Potential Hires to
Shadow a High-Performing Nurse

When you ask your interviewee to shadow one of your best nurses (clinically and professionally competent), that nurse can observe for any sign of rudeness or incivility. If left to spend a few hours or an entire shift with front line staff, people tend to let their guards down, at least a little. It may be enough to get a glimpse of their true personalities.

One manager had a male interviewee spend time with a high-performing male nurse on her unit. This potential hire had aced the interview, was well educated, and extremely polite with the female manager. After spending a few hours with the nurse on the unit, however, his great disposition began to unravel. He made two comments about "hot young nurses," and walked out of a patient's room to ask a nursing assistant to put his patient on a bedpan. When the nurse on staff asked him why, the potential hire said, "Well, isn't that her job?" This potential hire also casually dropped the f-bomb in the break room.

Do you think the staff member recommended this candidate for the job? Do you think the manager hired him? Not a chance. Having this potential hire shadow a competent and trusted nurse saved the manager from a bad hire and all the headaches that come with it.

Once I adopted this multi-pronged strategy, I starting consistently hiring good people while avoiding the bad. I remember once interviewing a candidate named Lisa for a nursing assistant position and thinking, right from the beginning, that she wouldn't be a good fit. She seemed to be apathetic, inarticulate, and just not right for our unit. Since I no longer relied solely on my own opinion, I went through the process of a staff interview and shadow. My staff loved Lisa! Based on their collective recommendation, I hired her, and Lisa turned out to be the most competent, compassionate, committed person on the unit.

HWF BEST PRACTICE TIP

BEHAVIORAL EXPECTATIONS

I've worked the term "behavioral expectations" into my new hire checklist. Not only do I cover the basics regarding timeliness and calling out, but I lay out the expectation of professionalism. It also lets a new hire know that bullying is not okay, and it needs to be reported immediately.

Cristina Suarez, Nurse Manager, Nicklaus Children's Hospital

When you're interviewing someone, you're not meeting him or her, you're meeting that person's representative. Spend more time up front making sure you bring in the right people and avoid hiring the wrong ones. Remember, once you get them in, it's hard to get them out!

HOW TO HANDLE THE CLINICALLY COMPETENT BUT TOXIC EMPLOYEE

Given that I travel 45 out of 52 weeks in a year, I spend a lot of time in airports. Often, when a flight is almost ready to leave, I'll hear the gate agent announce the names of the passengers who haven't yet boarded. "Gannon, party of three. Please proceed to gate A2 for immediate departure," etc. When I hear this, I say a simple prayer that they make

135

it! I've missed flights by just a few minutes and know what it's like!

A few years ago, I was at the Pittsburgh airport heading out to speak at a conference. As I sat at my gate, I heard a Southwest Airlines gate agent announce the names of four folks who hadn't yet boarded. Two minutes later, she announced their names again. And two minutes later, again. Finally, after announcing their names for a third time, I heard her say this, "Look, (said their names), we love you but we will leave you if you're not here in 30 seconds." You heard laughter among those of us who heard this announcement.

We love you but we will leave you. This mindset is perfect for front line managers when it comes to bullying and incivility. Taking this mindset to its logical conclusion can be tough, especially when you have a nurse on the unit who is extremely competent clinically but still toxic to those who work with him or her. This is especially true when there is a shortage of nurses or you have a lot of novice nurses in your unit.

To continue having the privilege of caring for patients, *every* employee needs to be clinically *and* professionally competent! Leaders need to set behavioral expectations in addition to clinical expectations and adopt the "love but leave" mindset. Leaders need to be tough on standards and expectations but tender with their people.

It's foolish to assume that a clinically competent nurse on your unit knows she is toxic. She may have received so many accolades for her clinical performance that she doesn't even realize there's a problem. She can't fix something if she doesn't know it's broken. It's your job to tell her.

Start by scheduling a private meeting, telling this nurse that you want to talk to her about something that is uncomfortable for you to say and may be uncomfortable for her to hear. Tell her that you need to be honest with her about her behavior. That although she is clinically competent, the way she treats people is not okay.

In your conversations, use key statements, such as the following:

- *The way you've been treating your coworkers is not okay.*

- *You are incredibly competent, and I also need you to step up and act in a professional manner.*

- *This is a professional environment, yet you have not been treating your coworkers professionally.*

Give examples and be as specific as possible. Let her know how her behavior impacts the work, patients, and each other. Here is an example:

> *Yesterday, when Mr. Rossi coded, you pushed Maggie out of the way and said, "Oh please, like you know what you're doing (in a sarcastic tone of voice). Let me handle this if you want him to live." This was a missed opportunity for you to support and coach Maggie—not criticize and humiliate her. I've seen you treat your coworkers as if they were incompetent many times before.*

Set Clear Behavioral Expectations

Setting expectations is an essential part of creating a professional workplace. Ideally, leaders should be setting those expectations right from the beginning, immediately upon hire. However, in situations in which a nurse has been wreaking havoc on the unit for decades but nobody's ever addressed it, you start now. As the Chinese proverb eloquently says, "The best time to plant a tree is 20 years ago. The second best time is now." Set behavioral expectations now.

Becky Calhoun is the director on a med/surg unit. She hired an experienced nurse whom she thought was an excellent hire. It wasn't before long that Becky started receiving complaints from her employees about her new "great" hire. Becky followed the process for addressing initial incidents of disruptive behaviors. She asked to meet with this nurse, used scripting techniques, "I'm not sure you're aware…. It's been brought to my attention…." and then provided her with a copy of the department norms. They engaged in a conversation about her coworker's perspectives, which resulted in dramatic improvements. Here is how Becky tells the story:

> A new, experienced nurse started on the unit. My staff were mentioning concerns with attitude and condescending behavior. I sat down with this nurse and went over the department norms agreement and explained the expectations of how we interact with each other and how the other staff members perceived her. This nurse admitted that she came from a place where people just were not that "nice." and she was not used to behaving respectfully. She thanked me for letting her know and told me she would im-

prove immediately. Since that conversation, the nurse has gotten along with staff well and became an engaged member of the team with no behavioral concerns. Staff members have positively commented on her actions, and the nurse herself emailed me to thank me again for giving her the opportunity to change.

Let's assume you realize that it's time to set behavioral expectations for Janine, a long-term nurse on the unit. First, get very specific about her behaviors and why others refer to her as toxic or "beastly." Make a list of everything she does that you believe is unprofessional and inappropriate. For example,

- Yells at someone for sitting in "her" chair

- Refuses to take report from certain nurses that she feels are beneath her

- Changes assignments when she doesn't like hers

- Openly criticizes her coworkers in front of others, even in patients' rooms

- Uses profanity in the nurses' station, hallways, and break rooms

- Sets new nurses up for failure by giving them the worst assignments

Then tell Janine you never want to witness these behaviors or hear about them ever again. Tell her how you expect her to behave and what the consequences are if she doesn't comply. Remind Janine that although you will give her the time to adapt her behavior, you're going to need to see immediate improvements.

Then tell Janine, "This is how we treat each other in this space" and be specific.

I expect you to …

- *Treat all chairs, computers, work stations, etc. as shared property.*

- *Take report from every nurse because patients' lives depend on a thorough report.*

- *Accept the assignment you've been given without causing a scene.*

- *Refrain from yelling, openly criticizing, or berating your coworkers in any public area.*

- *Avoid using any profanity in this organization.*

- *Support new nurses as they learn and grow by setting them up for success.*

Now, you may need to elaborate on these expectations a bit, but you get the point. Tell Janine the behaviors you no longer want to see and the behaviors you expect to start seeing. Spell it out so that she can't say she didn't understand.

Once you've had the honest conversation with Janine about her behavior and set behavioral expectations, one of two things is going to happen: She is going to step up and do the right thing or she is going to step out— either by quitting or by getting fired. That means you need to be willing to let Janine go if she doesn't step up.

According to Robert Sutton's book, *The No Asshole Rule: Building a Civilized Workplace and Surviving One That Isn't,* once you make the courageous decision to terminate a toxic employee, the remaining employees initially act as though they've just come out of 10 years of solitary confinement. They're not sure what that big bright light is in the sky; they meander around not really knowing which direction to go. However, once they realize they've been released from their prison, they step up and, like marshmallows in a cup of hot cocoa, rise to the top.

One nurse manager, after implementing the recommendations in this chapter, shared a story of culture change:

> The environment had been described as toxic by two nurses. It does not feel that way anymore, and employee retention has improved. I feel that hiring the right people is one of the most important things a manager can do, and now that all employees are trained, I continue to work for buy-in. I am trying to get staff involved in continuous improvement projects, councils, and leading huddles. These things were impossible six to eight months ago when it felt like I was doing everything I could just to keep the ship afloat.
>
> I find work challenging and exciting now, whereas I found it to be a burden and dreaded facing some days in the early spring. We all have a lot of work to do with how we communicate honestly and respectfully, but we are mindful and vigilant of that now and know we have to stay on top of it or the incivility can start creeping back.

Stop rationalizing, justifying, and ignoring toxic employees no matter how great they are clinically! You will never create a nurturing, supportive, and healthy workforce until you give equal weight to behavior.

We are hemorrhaging really great nurses to bullying and incivility. Like the gate agent for Southwest Airlines, "love" your people always but be willing to "leave" them if they don't hop on board in a timely fashion.

Holding your employees accountable for their behavior isn't just the right thing to do for your organization; it's the right thing to do for your employees and the patients you serve. It takes courage to therapeutically extract your most competent nurse because of behavior. It's easier to ignore or justify his or her behavior. However, as the leader, it's time to raise the bar. By holding everyone accountable for professional behavior and having the courage to remove someone, even a clinically competent provider, you're setting a higher standard.

As leaders in healthcare, we need to do better—and now that you're equipped with the strategies to engage in honest conversations with your employees, set behavioral expectations and now hold them accountable, you will do better!

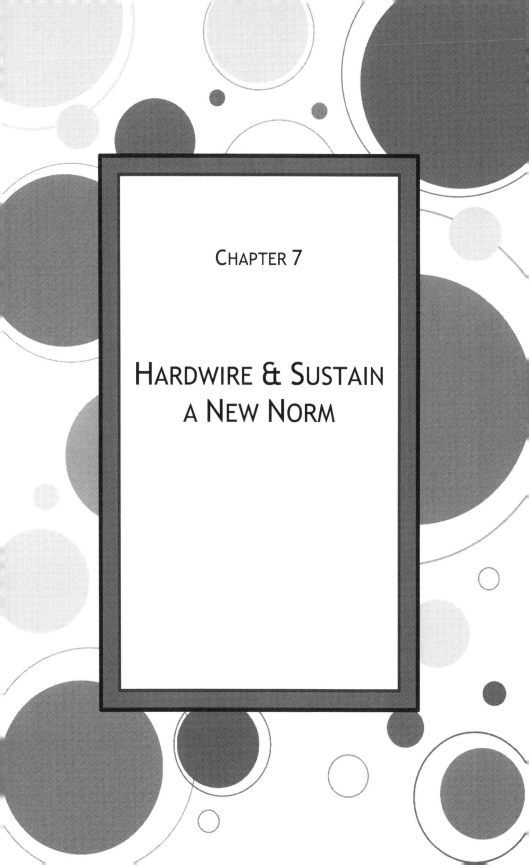

CHAPTER 7

HARDWIRE & SUSTAIN A NEW NORM

It takes time to create excellence. If it could be done quickly, more people would do it.

~ John Wooden

CHAPTER 7

HARDWIRE AND SUSTAIN A NEW NORM

When she accepted the position of manager, Theresa had no idea how dysfunctional the radiology department was. The department had the lowest morale scores of any in the organization, embarrassing People Survey scores, and turnover was 50%. Theresa needed help.

After adopting the process for addressing disruptive behaviors by setting expectations; holding people accountable; and cultivating a professional, supportive, and nurturing work environment, Theresa saw improvement. In just six months, morale increased and turnover dropped to 10%. However, Theresa didn't realize just how well the culture change was succeeding until she overheard an exchange between employees.

One of her nurses got "testy" with one of the techs, who replied, "Oh no. We don't play that game here anymore. Let's talk about this like professionals."

Theresa felt as if she exhaled for the first time in six months.

Changing a culture from bullying, incivility, and unprofessionalism doesn't happen overnight, but it does happen.

When key messages are repeated consistently over time, incidents of disruptive behavior are addressed immediately, and leaders keep their focus on the vision they created, culture change occurs.

When you think about it, isn't the ultimate goal of any leader to cultivate a culture where the team immediately rejects any incident of bullying and incivility; where professionalism becomes the new norm; where employees expect to receive direct feedback from their peers when they've been disrespectful or have made a mistake; where people talk *to* each other—not *about* each other, and where all employees speak up if they witness incidents of disruptive behavior?

As a leader, you reach this goal by "dripping" healthy workforce best practices into everyday practice, until they become the new norm. You want the norm to become hardwired into your culture.

In this chapter, we'll explore:

- How to consistently and frequently communicate expectations for professionalism

- How to build meaningful relationships with your employees

- How to make continuous learning an expectation and a habit

CONSISTENTLY AND FREQUENTLY COMMUNICATE EXPECTATIONS

Changing a culture by addressing disruptive behaviors requires repeated and consistent messaging over time, what I call a "drip campaign." While we most often see drip campaigns employed in business as a marketing strategy, the concept applies nicely to culture change.

You cannot introduce the topic of professional and respectful behavior once at a staff meeting and expect your employees to get it. Reminders of expected behavior need to be weaved into everything you do until appropriate behaviors become the new norm. And even then, the new norm needs to be maintained.

Numerous studies indicate the importance of repeating your key messages. In his book *The Advantage: Why Organizational Health Trumps Everything Else in Business,* Patrick Lencioni encourages leaders to over communicate clarity. Employees won't trust or believe any new message, focus, or change unless they've heard it at least seven times. This is especially true when it comes to communicating a change in expectations of how people treat each other. The following tactics will help you in hardwiring your message.

> HWF BEST PRACTICE TIP
> HEALTHY WORK ENVIRONMENT
> Have a "Healthy Work Environment" section in the unit's monthly newsletter that includes some tips, valuable information, or a positive quote.
> *Michelle Santello-Hunt MSN, RN, CNOR, Nurse Director, Jefferson Health New Jersey*

To hardwire the principles of a healthy workforce into the culture of an organization, it's critical to integrate healthy workforce topics into established meetings as a standing agenda item.

When I ask leaders how often they meet with their staff as a group, many admit that while the goal is to meet monthly, they're lucky if they meet twice a year. I get it. It's hard to carve out the time to consistently meet with a group of people, especially if you're a 24/7 shop. Getting the group together means your night staff may have to stay late or come in on their day off; your day staff may have to interrupt patient care to come to the meeting; or you'll have to repeat the same meeting several times to capture all of your employees.

There are many, many excuses why we don't meet regularly with our employees as a group. However, face time with your team is essential to set and reinforce behavioral expectations, communicate changes within the organization, and strengthen the bond among employees. If you're not regularly meeting with your staff, you're missing a key opportunity to build and sustain a cohesive team.

If you're not currently holding staff meetings, start small and start now. Just begin to schedule 30-minute meetings starting next month. If you are regularly meeting with your employees, kudos! You have an opportunity to kick it up a notch.

The agenda for your staff meetings should follow a consistent format, at least most of the time. I recommend the following:

1. **Celebrations**

   Ask your staff, "Is anyone celebrating anything this week/month?" Recognizing achievements and life events provides a great relationship-building opportunity because the employees get to know each other a bit beyond knowing only their birthdays.

Someone might say that she just got her acceptance letter to get her advanced degree, or that her daughter just had a baby. Someone else might share that he took a certification exam and passed, or that his son was just accepted to college. These little celebrations help build relationships and improve morale.

Note: If you know one of your employees achieved something important, use the meeting as an opportunity to recognize that individual in front of his or her peers.

I remember receiving a local award that was highlighted in our local paper and magazine as well as in the local news! I thought my manager would certainly mention my award at the next staff meeting, but she never said a word about it. Even though I am driven by an internal desire to accomplish and achieve, I felt deflated and unimportant. My manager missed the opportunity to acknowledge a member of the team who had achieved something. (And yes, she knew about the award.)

Don't miss an opportunity to recognize your employees' accomplishments, however small. Even if the accomplishment is running their first 5K!

2. Healthy Workforce

Use this portion of the meeting to reinforce behavioral expectations, acknowledge improvements, and "drip" education regarding professional behavior. I recommend you share an article, tip sheet, or show a video, and then open the meeting for discussions.

For example, one of the leaders in my *Eradicating Bullying & Incivility* course showed a four-minute clip about gossip from my video series "Coffee & Conversations about Nurse Bullying," and then asked the group, "Is gossip happening in our department?" Based on the looks on their faces, it was clear to all that gossip was an issue. She then asked:

- *How are we addressing this?*

- *Where should gossip never occur? (nurses' station, patients' rooms, patient care hallways, etc.)*

- *What actions do we need to take next?*

- *What can we do to speak more directly to each other instead of talking about each other behind our backs?*

- *How can we be better?*

The employees participated in the conversation and left the meeting agreeing to first protect patient care areas from any negative gossip. Over time, the leader noticed a decrease in the idle chitchat gossiping she had known was happening. Even the conversations people were having at the nurses' station changed!

3. **Overall Department Performance**
Sharing data about how the department is performing is important. Still, when the leader starts with the metrics the group did not achieve, it can feel like a lecture from a disappointed parent. Instead, flip the order around. Start with the metrics on which the group is doing well, followed by the opportunities for improvement. When sharing data

that falls below the goal, state the facts, but then say, "I know we can do better than this—that we are better. What's one thing we can do to improve this?"

I once worked for a manager who started every staff meeting with a list of our failures, the quality scores we didn't meet, the number of falls we had that month, turnover, etc. As each meeting started, I braced myself for what was to come. I came to dread these meetings just as everyone else did, including the manager!

If you're not meeting your metrics, ask your staff, "What's one thing we could do well that would have the greatest positive impact on this number?" Then be quiet and let them talk. Staff meetings need to be interactive, exploratory, and educational. Your employees should actually look forward to the meetings, not dread them like so many employees do.

4. **Organizational Updates**
   Finish the meeting with quick updates about any new organizational updates or changes.

HWF BEST PRACTICE TIP

OBSERVED BEHAVIOR

Present a case study or observed behavior (without names) to the employees at a staff meeting for discussion. Ask questions and listen to the answers. For example, was this behavior appropriate, given the situation? What was the problem with the scenario? How might it have been handled differently?

Michelle Santello-Hunt MSN, RN, CNOR, Nurse Director, Jefferson Health New Jersey

BUILD MEANINGFUL RELATIONSHIPS WITH EMPLOYEES

I was conducting a focus group with nurses who had less than one year's experience at an organization to determine how prevalent "nurses eating their young" was. I asked questions about relationships: the relationships the nurses have with their coworkers, the physicians, and their bosses. One nurse, who had been working on her unit for nine months, shared a disappointing story. Recently, this nurse overheard her manager talking with their unit-based educator. When the educator mentioned this nurse's name, the manager said, "Who's that?"

This nurse said, "I couldn't believe she didn't know who I was." I later found out that this nurse had already applied for another job in a different organization.

The studies conducted by Gallup about the importance of employee–boss relationships are widely known. According to Gallup, the number one reason someone stays or leaves his or her job is the relationship that individual has with his or her boss. The second reason has to do with whether or not that person feels a sense of belonging. Think about it—these are social reasons that have nothing to do with the benefits, types of patients, or location.

If you truly want to cultivate and sustain a professional, supportive, and nurturing workforce culture, building a relationship with your employees is mission critical. One strategy to build a relationship is to schedule regular one-on-one meetings with each employee.

HWF BEST PRACTICE TIP

BEGIN MEETINGS WITH SOMETHING POSITIVE

Brain science tells us that when you start a meeting with something positive, it influences the brains of the people in the meeting to be more positive for the next few hours.

Begin every meeting with something positive. Share a positive comment a patient shared about an employee. Pull out one of the commitments on your professional practice agreement and share a story of how an employee honored that commitment. Read a positive quote or affirmation. It almost doesn't matter what you share as long as it's positive.

Meeting with individual employees in a one-on-one forum is critical to establishing a healthy workforce. The challenge in healthcare is to carve out time consistently to meet with employees across multiple shifts and schedules, in the face of ongoing, unpredictable patient-care demands. Although these challenges may take precedence over employee meetings in a given moment, the key is to make one-on-one meetings an equal priority. Once employees trust that their leaders value time with them in addition to patients and unit functions, they will be more engaged and involved in creating and sustaining a healthy work culture.

How often you meet with your employees depends on how many direct reports you have. If you have more than 50 employees and you are the only leader, meeting quarterly with each employee is reasonable. If, however, you have less than 50 employees and/or have an assistant manager, you can meet more frequently, perhaps once per month. Please note that an employee's annual performance review does not count as a one-on-one.

You may think that it's impossible to meet with your employees monthly or even quarterly. However, best practice recommends meeting with employees weekly! These meetings do not need to take a lot of time, especially once you start meeting consistently.

To prepare for these meetings, spend time thinking about each employee and then categorizing them in your mind (not your records) according to the following three categories:

1. High Performers
    High performers are employees who cause you to breathe a sigh of relief when you learn they are working. They are competent at what they do and are role models for professional behavior. You never have to remind these nurses that their license is about to expire or that they need to complete their annual competencies. You've never had to engage in a conversation with them about their disruptive behavior. They step up consistently by getting involved in department improvements; are well respected by the physicians, support staff, and patients; and families love them.

    A common mistake leaders make is putting a nurse in the high-performing category just because she is clinically competent. You can't identify someone as a high performer if she is extremely competent but is mean and nasty. If this is the case, she is either "on the fence" or could be a low performer, depending on the severity of the toxicity.

2. On-the-Fence Performers
These nurses may be competent but do not always behave in a respectful manner. One of my clients talked to me about his charge nurse who was extremely competent and, in general, behaved professionally. She was the cheerleader when new employees started and the one who would organize employee birthday parties as well as baby and wedding showers. However, when stressed, this nurse would bark orders at people, occasionally throw things, and yell at her coworkers. After the crisis was over, she would apologize, but at the next crisis she would behave the same way.

I would consider this nurse an on-the-fence employee. She's competent but not always a professional role model.

3. Low Performers
Sometimes I refer to these people as "bottom dwellers." I keep bottom dweller in my mind, of course, never in an official employee document.

I know the term sounds harsh. However, if you look up the definition, bottom dwellers are people of low character, selfish, conniving, and without scruples. When you hear the word toxic, these are the employees that come to mind. They are the staff members who keep you up at night, that you worry about when you're not there, or who you know are undermining you and sabotaging others. These employees are the reasons why some of your good employees leave.

The problem is, at least sometimes, these nurses are your most competent staff members. If they weren't, you would have found a way to therapeutically extract them a long time ago.

Adopt a One-on-One Strategy

Once you've categorized your staff, schedule meetings with your high performers first. Why? Because they are the easiest to do and will help ease you into consistently conducting one-on-ones. If you start with your low performers first, you might feel the life being sucked out of you and be reluctant to schedule any more one-on-ones.

You may find that you only have a small handful of high performers! Not to worry; over time the goal will be to move some of your on-the-fence folks into the high-performing category!

When you meet with your high performers, just say this:

I think you're a superstar here. Any time I know you're working, I breathe a sigh of relief because you consistently make decisions based on what's best for our patients and what's best for our team. I just wanted you to know. Is there anything I can do for you?

That's it, at least during this first session. High performers are already motivated internally to perform well. They may have intrinsic reasons for showing up every day ready for practice despite the challenges. They don't need you to motivate them. However, they do need you to recognize how awesome they are.

Meet with your low performers next. The reason is because, like with the high performers, these meetings should be short and to the point. Your conversation is about setting clear expectations with them, as we talked about in Chapter 5. Provide these employees with specific behaviors you never want to see from them again and what you expect moving forward. This is critical.

For example, say this:

You are one of the most competent nurses in this department. However, the way you treat your coworkers is not okay.

It's been brought to my attention numerous times that you refuse to take report from nurses you don't like, and that when you're in charge, you give your friends the easy assignments and the nurses you don't like the more difficult ones.

These are behaviors I never want to see from you again. Period.

If you've created your department norms, give them a copy and go through where they are violating the agreement. Be clear and be serious. After the meetings, watch your low performers for any indication they are violating these expectations.

Lastly, meet with your on-the-fence employees. The reason that you meet with them last is because they may take more time. They need more coaching from you and support to improve. For these employees, you always want to acknowledge the strengths they bring to the department and what they could do better.

For example,

You're a competent and respectful charge nurse (add a specific action or competence that validates this statement). *However, when the department is under stress, you get reactive by throwing things and yelling at your coworkers, which then creates more stress for everyone. This is something I want you to work on. I'm willing to help you as long as you are willing to work on this.*

One of the leaders I worked with during a deep dive adopted the one-on-one strategy with a competent nurse who was often uncivil to her peers. During the meeting, he was honest with her (you're extremely competent but the way you treat people is not okay). She left his office tearful, but then after a few days, she thanked him for being honest with her and vowed to do better. A few months later, the leader sent me the following note:

> One of my nurses at the top of the list of incivility has really shown great improvement. After a conversation early in the spring, she became more aware of how she was coming across. She really put a lot of effort into thinking about what she was going to say prior to saying it. She spearheaded a welcoming project for new hires in which she gave them welcoming "goody bags" and posted signage welcoming them to the unit. One of the newer hires who had previously fallen victim to incivility at the hands of this nurse came and told me of the remarkable turnaround that this nurse has made.

Meeting one-on-one with your employees can be a game changer!

As I've worked with leaders who've adopted the one-on-one strategy, I find the following three questions/comments are the most powerful:

1. *What matters most to you right now?*

2. *Here is something you're doing well* (and be specific).

3. *Here is something I want you to work on* (and be specific).

Asking, "What matters most to you right now?" conveys interest, importance, and value to the employee. It shows that you care and genuinely want to know what's important to him or her. You may learn that one employee really wants an opportunity to advance. Another may care most about having a consistent schedule and getting out on time because young children are waiting at home. Hearing the answer to this question is especially valuable when the employee is different from you for any number of reasons. For example, if you are a baby boomer, you might be surprised by what's most important to one of your millennial nurses.

In the focus groups I facilitate, new nurses consistently complain that they have no idea how they're doing. One nurse said, "I don't know if I'm doing a good job or a bad job. Nobody tells me anything." I respectfully encourage every new nurse to ask for feedback, not to passively wait for someone to deliver it. However, it's also the leader's job to provide ongoing positive and constructive feedback to each employee in a way that helps the employee to continuously improve.

By saying, "Here is something you're doing well," you're reinforcing positive behaviors. You're letting your employee know what skills and behaviors he or she is doing well so those behaviors will be repeated. For example, when I was a new nurse, I loved drawing blood. It was fun for me. Over time, I became really good with a needle but didn't recognize that it was an admired skill until one of the more experienced nurses said to me, "Did anyone tell you how good you are with needles compared to some other nurses?" I was overjoyed. I knew I liked drawing blood gases and inserting IVs, but I didn't know that I excelled until that nurse acknowledged it. Once I realized this, I started offering to help other nurses either perfect IV insertion or blood draws, or would just do it for them.

One of my managers was the one to tell me that I was born to be an educator. She had heard me numerous times educating patients on new onset Afib, CAD, or new medications, and noticed that I had a way of explaining something complex and simplifying it, not only to patients but to other nurses! When she pointed this out to me, I started seeing myself as an educator and, sure enough, many years later, I went back to school and got my master's degree in nursing education.

Identify the strengths in each employee. Tell them. Don't assume they know. It's so much easier to tell people what they're good at than where they need to improve, isn't it? For some of us, giving constructive criticism can be so painful that we avoid those conversations completely. However, by avoiding the conversation, you're missing a huge opportunity to set a standard that, as a team, you are all on a path to continuous improvement. As with *kaizen*, the Japanese philosophy that focuses on continuous improvement, when you regularly provide feedback in this way, you convey an expectation that we all have something we need to work on.

To make it easier for you and your employee, present the constructive criticism as, "Here is one thing I want you to work on." By saying this, you're focusing on an area that needs to be improved and you're letting the employee know you are confident in his or her ability to work on it.

When the meeting is over, thank your employee and end with one of the following scripts:

> For high performers: *"<insert name>, I truly value you as a professional nurse here on <insert unit>."*

> For on-the-fence performers: *"I'm counting on you, <insert name>, to help create a more professional work environment here on <insert unit>."*

> For low performers: *"<insert name>, can I count on you to adhere to our professional practice agreement?"* (Or you may want to get very specific based on why you consider them a low performer).

HWF BEST PRACTICE TIP
SAY THE PERSON'S NAME

Every time you interact with an employee, say his or her name. Saying a person's name makes that person feel important. It's what I call the Nando Effect.

Every summer, some friends and I get together at a ski resort in western Pennsylvania. We stay in a beautiful cabin, eat, create amazing cocktails (I keep trying to like Bloody Marys but still can't bring myself to drink them!), and basically hang out at the pool all day and play games all night.

Every year the same core group of us goes, but we also invite other couples from time to time. One year, Bobbie, my graphic designer, and her soon-to-be husband at the time, Nando, joined us. This was the first time everyone met Nando, and I have to admit, anytime we bring in someone new, I worry slightly about upsetting the synergy of the weekend.

It didn't take long for everyone to fall in love with Nando. I observed him and figured out why it was so easy for everyone to accept Nando to the point where he became everyone's favorite by the time the weekend was over.

Every conversation Nando had with someone, including people he knew, such as my husband Ash and me, Nando said the individual's name.

- "Jenn, do you want another cup of coffee? How do you like your coffee, Jenn?"

- "Hey, Kim. Where did you get that recipe? … Kim, this chicken is so delicious."

- "Can you tell me more about your work, Luke? It sounds interesting. Tell me how you got started, Luke."

It wasn't overtly obvious that Nando kept saying someone's name. It was subtle, but it was there. By the end of the weekend, everyone loved Nando!

Saying someone's name out loud builds a relationship with that person. There is nothing sweeter to a human being than the sound of someone saying his or her name out loud. It makes us feel important.

Relationships are composed of micro moments of connection. Positive emotions compound quickly. To repeat myself, meeting one-on-one with your employees on a regular basis is a game changer. Not only does it give you the opportunity to provide both positive and constructive feedback, meeting regularly helps you to get to know your employees and allows your employees to get to know you.

HWF BEST PRACTICE TIP

HOW ARE YOU DOING TODAY?

Brain science shows that facing someone, looking that person in the eye, and asking, "How are you doing today?" increases the person's feelings of belonging. Every day, pick two to three employees to strengthen feelings of belonging. Approach each individually, look them in eye and ask, "How are you doing today?" as sincerely as possible.

MAKE CONTINUOUS LEARNING A HABIT—FOR YOURSELF AND YOUR EMPLOYEES

In Chapter 4, I mentioned that managing adult responsibilities didn't come easy for me. Thirty-some years ago, I was receiving food stamps, feeding my kids with government cheese and peanut butter, and scrounging for $5 to buy a book of stamps to pay my bills. It's true.

Like many young people, I made adult decisions with a teenager's pre-frontal cortex. I married at 19, became pregnant two months later, and because of pregnancy-related complications, quit college where I was enrolled in pre-med classes. My plan had been to become an OB-GYN physician. I wanted to deliver babies. My husband at the time (we eventually divorced) was young too and didn't know how to provide for a family.

My daughter was born, and then 10 months later I found out I was pregnant with my second daughter. I remember looking around at my tiny apartment, the empty refrigerator, and the calendar with the next date when I could pick up my supply of government cheese, and having that first *aha* moment. I was not living the life I expected or wanted. Right then, I decided that I wanted a better life for my kids. As a result, I went back to school to become a nurse. The journey from there to here wasn't easy, but 30+ years later, I can tell you that it was the best decision I've ever made.

If you asked me what made the biggest difference in my ability to go from eating government cheese and counting pennies to having a doctoral degree and a successful business, it was one simple action I took that day.

When I decided I wanted a better life for myself and for my kids, the first thing I did was take a trip to the library. There, I reactivated my card and borrowed the maximum, 10 books. I started reading books on personal development, finances, spirituality, relationships, and more.

It didn't happen instantly, but something started to shift in my brain. My mindset changed from being a passive observer to an active participant in my life. With my two girls and empty refrigerator in mind, I made a commitment to continuous learning. I haven't stopped learning since. My most valuable possession, other than my family and friends, is my library card.

If you want to reach your full potential and be known as an authentic leader who cultivates and sustains a high-performing, professional, and cohesive team, you must make continuous learning a habit. And, you need to stress the exact same thing with your employees—make ongoing learning about how employees treat each other an expectation of the job until it becomes a habit.

HWF BEST PRACTICE TIP
READ TO IMPROVE

I spend a minimum of 30 minutes each day reading something instructional or inspirational. I read books on organizational/team culture (just finished reading Patrick Lencioni's book, *Advantage*), books on human behavior (Robert Cialdini's book, *Influence,* is a winner), books to help me become a better business owner, and books to help me become a better human. I also read journal articles, online blogs, and listen to podcasts and CDs when getting ready in the morning or driving in my car.

I've made reading a habit and it's changed my life. I will go without food before I will go without reading. Reading is more nourishing.

You can't share one article, send your employees to a workshop on disruptive behaviors, or even set behavioral expectations, and then check a check box (Yep! Everyone should know how to behave now. Check.). Cultivating and sustaining a healthy, professional workforce culture requires ongoing training and education. However, teaching people doesn't necessarily have to be a big deal. What I have found works best and produces the greatest shifts in departments is when the leader incorporates small bits of content slowly over a period of time. Here are some ideas:

Establish a Healthy Workforce Bulletin Board

I mentioned posting articles on a Healthy Workforce Bulletin Board in Chapter 4. Hanging such a bulletin board in your employees' break room, frequently used conference room, or locker room is a simple way to keep healthy workforce top-of-mind. Wherever the majority of your employees gather is a good place, unless that's in a patient care area! (Patients and their families read everything in the hallways, especially if they're walking around out of boredom. Families may wonder why you need to go through the practice of creating a board and posting behavioral expectations in a professional environment!)

When decorating this board, make it fun yet professional. A leader in a pediatric hospital decorated her first board in a way that looked as if it could have been located in a kindergarten. This leader's initial thought was that the style fit that of the hospital's patients. But the board was not for the patients—it was for employees who are considered professionals. It's great to have fun with your board, but make sure it looks professional. Get your employees involved in designing the board. I've included a guide with a few examples in the Resource Vault. For access, go to https://theHealthyWorkforceInstitute.com/Resource-Vault/.

On your Healthy Workforce Bulletin Board, post your professional practice agreement (department norms), and any tip sheets, articles, positive affirmations, quotes, or messaging related to professional behavior. While some of what you post should be inspirational and positive, it's equally important to include content related to disruptive behavior. For example, I've created a survey called, "What if the bully is you?" It's appropriate to put this survey on the board and ask employees to take a copy and complete it. You can post a large envelop with a big note that says, "Take me." (For access to the survey, go to https://theHealthyWorkforceInstitute.com/Resource-Vault/

As a doctoral-prepared professional, I'm all about evidence-based practice. However, if you give me a 15-page article full of statistical analysis, variables, Cronbach's alpha testing, and *p* values, my eyes gloss over. Look for articles that your employees will read. If you find an article from *Forbes Online* about gossip, print the article and post it. If you read an editorial in a nursing journal about helping nurses articulate their value through improved communication with the interdisciplinary team, post it. Post any articles or stories you find about professionalism.

I've been writing a new blog article every week for the last eight years. I've won numerous awards for my blog, and I welcome you to go through the archives and post articles you find relevant to a healthy workforce culture. Just go to https://HealthyWorkforceInstitute.com/blog.

The key is to consistently share content related to improving yourselves as a team in a way that becomes a habit. In his book, *Atomic Habits: An Easy & Proven Way to Build Good Habits & Break Bad Ones,* James Clear shows us how incorporating tiny habits into our daily practice that result in a 1% improvement can transform our lives and deliver remarkable results. As the leader, your goal should be small improvements over time.

Make continuous learning a habit with your team. As I said earlier, this can be as simple as picking an article or video for your staff to read/watch, and then discussing the topic during a staff meeting.

However, knowing that staff meetings occur monthly at best, another way to inspire continuous learning and education is to continually post fresh articles, perhaps about assertive communication (honest and respectful). Let your employees know you've posted an article and that you want them to read it. Throughout the week during huddles, one-on-ones, or counseling or coaching sessions with an employee, bring the article up. Pull out a recommendation or strategy from the article and engage in a conversation with your employees.

When working with departments doing deep dive consulting, I begin by working with the team to establish department norms. The next step is to start focusing on monthly themes. Typically, I recommend starting with assertive communication for a month or two, and then choosing another topic, such as conflict resolution, positivity, or building a cohesive team, etc. Assertive communication is always an appropriate theme, but you can choose from a variety of topics relevant to your department. Here are just a few examples:

- Building trust
- Eliminating incivility
- Choosing open language
- Giving feedback
- Engaging in peer-to-peer accountability
- Understanding across generations
- Building positive relationships

Pick a topic you believe impacts the overall culture in your department. Then choose articles, affirmations, videos, etc. that provide nuggets of education on that topic. This enables you to immerse your employees in the topic slowly, over a course of a month, so that by the end of the month they've improved in that area. Even if the improvement is 1%, as James Clear suggested, the collective improvement in your team can be palpable.

While I've given you several tactics, you may feel a bit overwhelmed and unsure of how to actually operationalize these tactics. Not to worry. Here's how you can pull it all together into a simple plan:

Step 1: Pick a topic for the month

Step 2: Search for articles, tips, videos, etc. related to that topic

Step 3: Post an article or tip sheet once a week on your Healthy Workforce Bulletin Board (or staff communication board if you choose not to create a separate board)

Step 4: Let your employees know you've added something new

Step 5: Include that topic during your monthly staff meeting

Get yourself and your employees into a habit of always learning how to become better humans and a better team. As leadership guru John Maxwell is quoted as saying, "You don't necessarily need to instruct people over and over again, but you certainly need to remind them."

Cultivating a healthy workforce culture isn't an initiative that you can roll out once and expect for it to continue on its own. The principles we've talked about have to become embedded into the fabric of your department and reinforced often.

When you introduce your plan to build a healthy workforce culture, someone might ask, "How do we make sure this isn't just 'one more thing' in a sea of other important improvements?" Unfortunately, most employees can point to times when new programs were announced and then quickly faded. You can't change the past, but you can consistently bring healthy workforce concepts and principles to the agenda. Eventually, even your more skeptical employees will realize it's there to stay.

If treating each other with respect as professionals is important, you can *never* take it off the agenda in your meetings. In fact, you should express your expectations about professionalism and respect in interviews and keep right on going from there. When James Clear, the habit genius, is asked how long it takes to establish a habit, he always replies, "Forever. Because as soon as you stop practicing the habit, the habit goes away."

Once you've done the work of heightening awareness about bullying and incivility in the workplace and confronted it directly, you have a lot to be proud of. But don't stop there! The real culture change comes with hardwiring a culture of respectful and professional behavior. With time and patience, you can create that healthcare environment you imaged when you began this book.

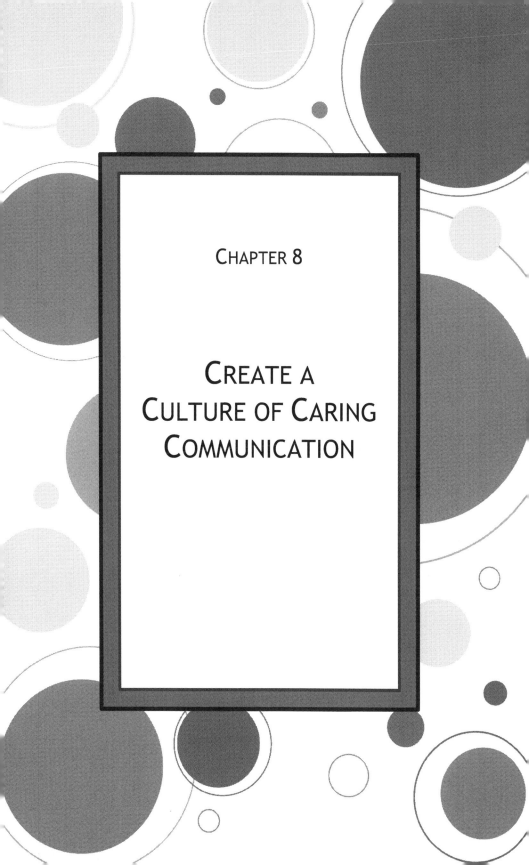

CHAPTER 8

CREATE A
CULTURE OF CARING
COMMUNICATION

Nurses need to extend the same compassion to each other as we do to our patients.

~Renee Thompson

CHAPTER **8**

CREATE A CULTURE
OF CARING COMMUNICATION

If you've been a nurse for any length of time, you are quite familiar with the ubiquitous ways nurses torture each other. The old eat their young; nurses get thrown under the bus in front of important people (sometimes patients); the day shift battles with the night shift; and, in a fate worse than death, nurses come to work only to find they have been pulled to another unit (where they'll be tortured).

Over the years, I've developed four initiatives to counter these and other painful situations:

1. Create sacred spaces within patient care areas.

2. Roll out the red carpet for float staff and travelers.

3. Set the next shift up for success.

4. Act as "mother bear" to new employees.

In this chapter, we'll explore each of these initiatives. Departments that have adopted these initiatives have transformed their cultures, resulting in a ripple effect of caring communication across their organizations. You can experience the same results.

CREATE SACRED SPACES IN ALL PATIENT CARE AREAS

Thousands of healthcare employees experience or witness incidents of bad behavior in the workplace perpetrated by their colleagues on a regular basis. These behaviors range from eye rolling and gossip to yelling, undermining, and sabotage. Out of all of the behaviors identified, the most common behaviors reported by healthcare employees are being yelled at, openly criticized, or mocked in front of others.

Unfortunately, many times one of the "others" is a patient or family member.

The following quotes represent just a few examples:

No matter how hard I try, Jackie always finds fault with how I leave my patients at the end of my shift. What makes it worse is that she berates me in front of my patients during shift report. It's so embarrassing!

The charge nurse barged into my patient's room while I was giving meds and yelled, "Elena called off again so now we're going to be short staffed yet again. You'll have to take another admission," and then stormed out of my room, leaving me to make an attempt to reassure my patient and his wife that although we were short, he would receive good care.

Patients frequently witnessed interactions between me and other nurses and asked, with concern, "Are you okay after what she said to you?" or "Sounds like she is having a really bad day," or "I felt really uncomfortable seeing that interaction, but most of all I feel bad for you."

I don't have to repeat how behaviors like these negatively impact nursing performance, employee well-being, patient satisfaction, and outcomes. One viable solution is to establish sacred spaces in all areas frequented by patients and their families.

A sacred space is one distinguished from all other spaces because of the rituals that are practiced within that defined space. Most commonly used for religious purposes, sacred spaces are usually identified by something physical, such as a temple or symbol, and a ritual-based practice that occurs within that space, such as prayer. But non-secular sacred spaces exist too.

You can't watch a sunrise, sunset, or a storm rolling across the sky with lightning, walk through the woods, or look down from a mountaintop without feeling the magnitude of nature. Nature is the equalizer for all people and all things made by humanity. In nature we truly sense the presence of something more, a higher power. Nature is our first sacred space—before religious temples and churches.

Men have "man caves" that are never to be violated by lavender scented candles, lace, or Kenny G soft jazz. Sometimes the sacred spaces for women are their bathtubs because that's the only space others, especially their kids, won't invade! But many of us have a special place in our homes that we protect from disruptions.

My daughter found an amazing place to get pedicures in Raleigh, North Carolina, where she lives. I live in Pittsburgh, Pennsylvania, and when I visited her shortly after this discovery, my daughter insisted we get pedicures. We started chatting as soon as we sat in the chairs. Immediately, we got the "Shhhh! This is a sacred space," from the nail specialists, who then pointed to a sign that read: To experience our calming and relaxing pedicures, we ask that you respect this sacred space by turning off your phones and refraining from talking. Best relaxing pedicure ever!

Sacred spaces are everywhere if you just look for them, and, without a doubt, sacred spaces should exist in healthcare too.

A patient's room is the ultimate sacred space and the one that should be most protected. Violating this space should be a never event, yet it's surprising how often bad behavior happens in a patient's room. It's not okay.

The hallways in front of patient rooms also need to be kept sacred. Patients and their family members hear everything. What you say in the hallways filters directly into the patients' rooms. Remember the story about a nursing assistant who threatened a nurse in the hallway, saying, "My boyfriend knows what shuttle you take and is going to be waiting for you to beat the sh** out of you!"? A patient's wife was the one who reported that incident. Imagine how she felt about that nursing assistant caring for her husband!

Another area to keep sacred is the nurses' station. Again, patients and their family members hear everything! For some reason, nurses think there is an invisible force field surrounding the nurses' station which blocks sound from leaking out. Wrong. Not only do patients hear nurses talking, they actively try to listen to the conversations in case the medical team is talking about them!

What if you work in an ambulatory care setting, such as an outpatient dialysis clinic? Your entire department can't be a sacred space, right? Wrong! If your outpatient clinic or department is an open area where patients receive care, the answer is "yes." Your entire department *is* a sacred space!

A critical care nurse told me how a surgeon responded when she was late bringing a patient down to the OR. In front of the patient, the surgeon said, "Why are you so late? If this patient dies on the table, it's your fault!"

Creating sacred spaces for your patients and their family members is not only the right thing to do for them, it's the right thing to do for you and your colleagues. We get so caught up in our work we sometimes forget that healthcare is a service industry in which we are called to serve our public and each other. By honoring and defending the spaces where we intimately care for our patients, we demonstrate the respect for the one sacred and precious life we each have.

ROLL OUT THE RED CARPET FOR FLOAT STAFF AND TRAVELERS

One of the most-anxiety provoking situations for employees is to come into work and find out they have been pulled to another unit for their shift. Why? Because employees who get pulled are usually treated like gum on someone's shoe.

Float staff, agency, and travelers frequently receive the worst patient assignments. We exclude, ignore, and torture them. I've heard nurses say, "Well, travelers and agency nurses make the big bucks, they should expect to get the worst patients." Imagine any of the following happening to you:

You get pulled to another unit where they won't give you the code to the staff bathroom. You have to leave the unit and find a public bathroom.

You get pulled to another unit where the staff hides the blood pressure cuffs and won't give you a med cart.

As an agency nurse, you are regularly assigned all the isolation, incontinent, and dementia patients.

Why do nurses treat people who are there to help them so horribly? Is it because they make more money? If their mom were a patient on their unit, would they still give someone who has never worked on their unit before and who might not be fully knowledgeable about caring for their patient population the worst assignments just because they make a few more bucks? Does it make nurses feel superior to be able to look down on someone else? Do nurses feel they've earned their stripes in the school of hard knocks and want to make sure no one else gets off easy?

Rolling out the red carpet means you treat all people who don't normally work on your unit (float staff, agency, travelers, etc.) like guests in your home. By rolling out the red carpet, you demonstrate the respect all humans deserve, and patients ultimately receive better care.

Treat anyone who is providing a service on your unit like a celebrity, as someone extraordinary who deserves special treatment. You can make a huge difference in that person's work experience and the care delivered to your patients simply by going out of your way for a service provider.

To begin making this change on your unit or department, gather as many employees as you can during a staff or ad hoc meeting. Name the initiative, "Red Carpet Treatment," and ask employees to identify ways they can treat floaters and agency employees like guests in their home. Rolling out the red carpet could be as simple as asking employees who have been pulled in the past what made for a good experience and what made for a bad experience. The key is to engage everyone in the process!

If you are the manager on a unit that has a floater, pay special attention to that person and situation. Introduce yourself as the leader, welcome the person, and thank him or her for being there. Throughout the day, check in and ask how things are going. Make sure you follow up with the individual's home unit manager (if the person got pulled to your unit) or with the individual's agency to get feedback about the experience. As the leader, you should actively seek feedback about a floater's experience.

If one of your employees gets pulled to another unit, make sure you stop by at some point during the day. Ask how things are going and remind the person how much he or she is helping the other employees on that unit. It is critically important to get feedback—good, bad, or ugly—and share that feedback with the manager on the receiving unit. Do so in the spirit of continuous improvement.

Nobody likes to find out that someone had a bad experience on his or her unit. If this happens to you, try not to get defensive. Try to see it as an opportunity to improve everyone's experience, whether it's someone in the home unit, pulled, a traveler, or a nurse from an agency, etc. In the end, the way we treat each other reflects on your entire organization.

SET THE NEXT SHIFT UP FOR SUCCESS

Each shift seems to believe that they collectively do more than the other shift and that somehow the opposite shift has it easier. They forget that care happens over a 24-hour period. Although differences exist in the structures of the shifts, patients still get admitted; unexpected crises occur; and medication administration, assessments, and documentation occur day and night.

It's unclear why employees think their shift is the only shift that works hard. What is clear is that they respond by fighting with subtle, yet destructive, weapons. Employees of one shift fight with those of the other—not overtly. No. Their weapons are subtle but still lethal. Here are how some of the weapons work:

Dumping is when nurses deliberately leave work for the next shift. For example, they retime medications so they appear on the next shift; conveniently postpone that CT of the head scan for later; and somehow leave all of the patients' IV bags dry to the point where next shift nurses have to get all new tubing.

Nurses withhold information by "forgetting" to let the next nurse know that the physician wants to be paged as soon as the patient's wife arrives. The physician rounds later and discovers the wife has been there for over two hours. The physician berates the unknowing nurse.

One of the biggest battlefields in the shift war is shift report. This is where the nitpicky, condescending attitudes, micromanaging, and criticism occur. Some nurses are petrified to give report to certain nurses because of how those nurses treat them.

Nurses complain constantly about being short staffed. However, is the problem the number of nurses working or is it the behavior of the nurses? We have to stop this war with our counter shift. Ultimately, when you dump on the next shift, withhold information, and leave everything a mess, you're impacting their ability to provide good care to your patients.

To change your unit's culture from engaging in shift wars to setting each other up for success, gather the employees from your unit. Ask this question: How can you set the next shift up for success? Ask all employees for their input on what the previous shift could do to make it easier for the next shift to take the baton and run!

HWF BEST PRACTICE TIP
END THE SHIFT WARS

Cristina Suarez, a nurse manager at Nicklaus Children's Hospital, and her team wanted to end the "shift wars" on their unit. The unit council took Nurses Week celebrations as the opportunity to promote teamwork. Each day, depending on the theme, the previous shift would leave the staff lounge decorated and with some goodies for the oncoming shift to enjoy. It allowed the leaders to sit back and witness the staff doing nice things for the opposite shift. It made a huge difference in morale and was so much fun!

ACT AS MOTHER BEAR TO ALL NEW EMPLOYEES

Mother bears are the quintessential role models for loving and protecting their offspring. When a mother bear detects a threat to her cubs, she attacks! A mother bear will sacrifice her life to save her cubs.

When a cub cries out of hunger or discomfort, the mother bear feeds, warms, or moves the cub to dry land. When the cub yells because it can't find its mother, the mother grunts and returns to her cub. When the cub screams because it is in danger, the mother bear charges and attacks! The most dangerous place to be is between a mother bear and her cubs. We need to protect our new employees like a mother bear protects her cubs.

As you'll remember from earlier chapters, 25-33% of all new nurses quit annually and half of all graduating nurses are afraid they will become the target of workplace bullying.

Fortunately, you don't need to be female or the manager to be a mother bear. "Mother bear" is a mindset—not a gender. It's about doing everything you can to support and protect new employees, knowing how vulnerable they are.

Preceptors, of course, are the primary mother bears, but they don't always do the job well. For example, Annie was nervous about her first job as a new nurse and had trouble sleeping as she anticipated her first day. She didn't know who her preceptor was, so upon arrival to the unit, she stopped at the nurses' station. When the unit secretary looked up, Annie told the secretary her name and that she was new to the unit. The unit secretary looked on the schedule, found her name and hollered for Cindy who was to be her preceptor.

Cindy looked up at her from the desk, sighed, and gave a look of disgust. She motioned for the new nurse to come to where she was sitting. Cindy then told Annie, "Hey, I didn't want to be a preceptor, but they told me that I had to if I wanted to get a raise this year. So, you're stuck with me.

Try to stay out of my way and make sure you don't kill anyone on *my* shift!" Everyone around her laughed. Needless to say, Annie had been right to be afraid. Shame on this preceptor and everyone who laughed rather than support this new cub nurse. And shame on the leader who allows this attitude to reign in the unit.

Research conducted through the Vermont Nursing Partnerships resulted in a rich body of knowledge related to the integration of new nurses through their relationships with their preceptor and colleagues. The preceptor assumes many roles in helping to transition a new graduate nurse into professional practice. Roles such as *protector*, educator, socializer, evaluator, and role model provide a framework in which the preceptor can coach a new nurse. Preceptors, regardless of their gender, therefore, need to become the primary, but not the only, mother bears for new employees.

Did you know that black bear mothers stay with their cubs for 16-17 months? The family bond remains strong right up to the moment the cub leaves to start his or her own family. So remember that even after the preceptor orientation is over, the preceptor should continue to protect new nurses so they can grow into the strong, competent, and compassionate nurses we know they can be!

Welcoming new employees to your department shouldn't feel like a burden. It should feel like a joyous occasion, filled with hope, excitement, and optimism, just like any parent feels when bringing their child into the world. Celebrate your new people—don't eat them! Don't let anyone else eat them either!

It would be wonderful if we could simply establish healthcare environments as places where bullying and incivility were simply not tolerated. As a leader, you have the opportunity to do even more! You can build a culture of caring with the initiatives described in this chapter. Begin getting your team to designate sacred spaces, roll out the red carpet, set the next shift up for success, and act as mother bear to new employees. When they are busy doing these things, no one will be lining up at your office door to tell you their complaints. They will be using that time and energy to support each other and deliver exceptional care.

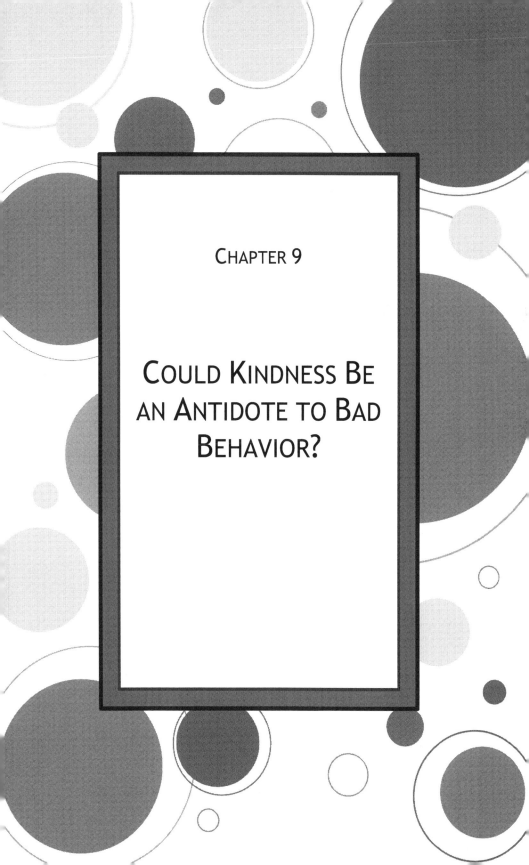

CHAPTER 9

COULD KINDNESS BE AN ANTIDOTE TO BAD BEHAVIOR?

Kind hearts are the gardens,
Kind thoughts are the roots,
Kind words are the flowers,
Kind deeds are the fruits,
Take care of your garden
And keep out the weeds,
Fill it with sunshine, Kind words, and Kind deeds.
~Henry Wadsworth Longfellow

CHAPTER 9

COULD KINDNESS BE AN
ANTIDOTE TO BAD BEHAVIOR?

When my daughters were young, they went trick or treating with the neighborhood kids while I stood at the front door handing out candy. I enjoyed watching the other kids run from house to house to get their tasty treats. Many parents tagged along, standing on the street as the kids ran from door to door, hoping to get a candy bar and not just a piece of Bit-O-Honey, or worse, an apple!

As I watched over the years, I noticed that even though the kids could take short cuts by running through their neighbors' yards, they didn't. They ran down the driveways, on the street a bit, and then up the next driveway. A few times, one rogue kid would attempt to take a shortcut through the rhododendrons, but a parent (any parent) quickly hollered and made the kid go back. Everyone knew it was considered rude if you ran through someone's front yard, especially in a nice neighborhood.

TIMES HAVE CHANGED

I rarely get to participate in Halloween now because of my travel schedule. My grown daughter, however, called me after her first experience with trick or treaters. "Mom!" she said, "Can you believe these kids just run from house to house through people's yards! You would have never let us do that. How rude."

DO YOU THINK RUDENESS IS ON THE RISE WITH KIDS?

Jean Twenge, a professor at San Diego University, says students are 30% more narcissistic than they were 25 years ago. Other experts agree. We could spend the rest of our time in this chapter talking about the reasons why (technology, lack of parental role modeling, limited supervision after school, etc.). The point is, rude kids can grow up to be rude adults.

Everywhere we look, it seems that disruptive behaviors are on the rise. The problem is certainly not limited to healthcare. Bad behaviors are showing up across the globe, in our cities, schools, neighborhoods, and homes. For example, I can hardly keep up with the reports of bad behavior on airplanes. Every day and everywhere, we witness or hear reports of acts of cruelty, ignorance, bullying, incivility, and just plain ol' meanness. We can just sit around complaining and share the horror on Facebook—or we can do something about it.

COULD KINDNESS BE AN ANTIDOTE?

We've spent most of our time together discussing how to eradicate bad behavior in healthcare. As we wrap up, let's explore the other side of the spectrum of human behavior—the good—a bit more. While this book focused on equipping you with the strategies and tactics leaders need to address bullying and incivility, the ultimate goal is for you to cultivate and sustain a healthy, professional, respectful, supportive, and kind workforce culture.

ONCE YOU'VE ADDRESSED THE BADNESS, IT'S TIME TO CULTIVATE THE GOODNESS

According to David Hamilton, a PhD prepared organic chemist who advocates for kindness in the workplace, spreading kindness provides compounding benefits in the workplace. Kindness isn't just a right brained, hippie, "let's hold hands together and sing kum ba yah" tactic. Neuroscience proves that in spreading a culture of kindness, you rewrite the story of your department.

Although elements that are brutal, cruel, and animalistic exist in humanity, we are actually hardwired to serve and help others. We get a biological reward when we extend kindness toward another human through the release of endorphins that produce a "helper's high." Our brains are equipped and ready to respond with a release of chemicals that reinforce kindness, collaboration, and cooperation with others. I repeat, despite what you see on the news and what might be happening in your department, humans are wired for kindness.

KINDNESS IS CONTAGIOUS

Being kind inspires others to be kind, creating a ripple effect. Like seed pods from a plant that the wind gently blows and scatters to neighboring yards, when we scatter kindness, we can watch it grow.

Paige Roberts and her team at the University North Carolina Chapel Hill implemented a "Scatter Kindness, Watch it Grow" campaign. This campaign encouraged acts of kindness among staff members. Staff placed a "dandelion seed" on a prominent unit bulletin board when they performed an act of kindness and a "dandelion flower" on the bulletin board when they received one. Over the initial six-week period, the board progressively filled up with a wide variety of acts of kindness, from a gift card to Starbucks to helping another staff member bathe a patient. These acts of kindness continue on. Paige said,

> Intentional efforts to increase positivity at work, including kindness, have resulted in improvements in every staff and patient outcome, including a stronger patient safety culture, increased staff resilience, and a significant decrease in staff turnover. These simple efforts truly can make a remarkable difference, even in the most stressful and chaotic healthcare environments.

As the leader in your department, you have an ethical responsibility to your organization, your employees, and the patients you serve to stop the badness. You know this and now you've been given the tools to be able to do that. Now will you join me on the path to cultivating kindness?

Here are some ways to get started:

- Find at least one opportunity today to thank a staff member for being nice. Watch how that person responds and how your praise affects his or her behavior toward others.

- During shift change or the end of the workday, ask your employees who are leaving to name three good things that happened during their work hours. If possible, do this in a group. By default, humans tend to focus on the negative; we're actually designed that way. However, by "forcing" them to identify three good things, it influences them to look for good things during their shift. If you do this consistently, over time you will experience less complaining and more celebrating.

- Set an expectation of kindness *before* you hire someone. Say these words in your next interview, "Kindness isn't optional here. It's a requirement of this job."

- Look for opportunities to praise your employees on a regular basis. According to a McKinsey global survey, praise from an immediate manager, attention from a leader, and opportunities to lead a project have more impact on motivation than do monetary incentives. Your employees complain about money, but they care more about the relationship they have with you.

- In your huddles, staff meetings, council meetings, etc., start by sharing three positive comments from patients, other departments, physicians, etc. By doing this, you influence the way your teams interact with others.

- Ask an employee whose attitude tends toward the negative for help with a project. This will help to engage the employee in a positive way.

As a reminder, your role as leader is more important and more influential than you think. Be the type of leader you would want to have.

I leave you with one final question: What can you do to cultivate and spread the goodness?

As the late Mr. Rogers so eloquently said, "When I was a boy and I would see scary things in the news, my mother would say to me, "Look for the helpers. You will always find people who are helping." Address the badness but look for the goodness. You will find it.

As I said in the beginning pages of this book, I don't want you or any nurse leader to experience what I did in my first job as a front line leader in healthcare. I am confident that you, like me, care about your staff and your patients at a profound level. You want to create a culture of professional and compassionate behavior in the best interests of both your employees and your patients. Chances are that until now you were never given the tools to do this. In fact, you entered a world where toxic behavior had been normalized—and were expected to function within it. Now you have the tools and strategies you need to confront the bad and introduce the good in your unit or department. You can create expectations and hold people accountable for professional behavior in the workplace. Use the tools and strategies, and I know you'll do a fantastic job in making your department a better place for everyone, employee or patient, who spends time there. Thank you for making the world of healthcare a better place.

END NOTES

END NOTES

CHAPTER 2

"2016 National Healthcare Retention & RN Staffing Report." *NSI Solutions* (2016).

Rosenstein, A., and O'Daniel, M. "A Survey of the Impact of Disruptive Behaviors and Communication Defects on Patient Safety." *The Joint Commission Journal on Quality and Patient Safety* (2008).

Kovner, C., Brewer, C.., Fatehi, F. and Jun, J. "What Does Nurse Turnover Rate Mean and What Is the Rate?" *Policy, Politics, & Nursing Practice* (2014).

Townsend, T. "Break the Bullying Cycle." *American Nurse Today* (2012).

Maxfield D., Grenny J., McMillan R., Patterson K., Switzler, A. "Silence Kills: The Seven Crucial Conversations for Healthcare." *American Association of Critical Care Nurses* (2005).

"Modern Nurse Survey." *RN Network* (2018).

"Workplace Bullying from the Perspective of U.S. Business Leaders." *Workplace Bullying Institute* (2013).

Physical and Verbal Violence Against Healthcare Workers. Sentinel Event Alert 2018. *The Joint Commission* (2018).

"Facts about the Magnet Recognition Program®." *American Nurses Credentialing Center [ANCC]* (2017).

Professional Issues Panel on Incivility, Bullying, and Workplace Violence. *American Nurses Association (ANA)* (2015).

Workplace Incivility, Lateral Violence and Bullying Among Nurses: A Review about Their Prevalence and Related Factors. *Act BioMed for Health Professions* (2018).

DOL Workplace Violence Program — Appendices. *U.S. Department of Labor.*

CHAPTER 3

"Violence, Incivility, and Bullying." *American Nurses Association* (2016).

Porath, C. *Mastering Incivility: A Manifesto for the Workplace* (2016).

"Civility in America: An Annual Nationwide Survey," Weber Shandwick (2016).

"The 'Dirty Dozen': 12 Persistent Safety Gaffes that We Need to Resolve." *Institute for Safe Medication Practices (ISMP)* (2014).

Workplace Bullying Institute 2017 National Survey.

CHAPTER 4

Useem, M. "Four Lessons in Adaptive Leadership," *Harvard Business Review* (2010).

Covey, S. *The 7 Habits of Highly Effective People* (2013).

Senge, P. *The Fifth Discipline* by Peter M. Senge (1990).

Towery, T. *The Wisdom of Wolves: Leadership Lessons from Nature* (2013).

CHAPTER 5

CareerBuilders with Harris Interactive© Survey (2012)

Sutton. R. *The No Asshole Rule: Building a Civilized Workplace and Surviving One That Isn't.* (2007)

CHAPTER 7

Lencioni, P. *The Advantage: Why Organizational Health Trumps Everything Else in Business* (2012).

Gallup State of American Workplace (2017).

Cialdini, R. *Influence: The Psychology of Persuasion* (1993).

Clear, J. Atomic Habits: *An Easy & Proven Way to Build Good Habits & Break Bad Ones* (2018)

CHAPTER 8

Boyer, S. "Competence and Innovation in Preceptor Development." *Journal of Nurses in Staff Development* (2008).

Dewhurst, M., Guthridge, M, and Mohr, E. "Motivating People: Getting Beyond money" McKinsey Quarterly (2009).

CHAPTER 9

Twenge, J. *Generation Me: Why Today's Young Americans Are More Confident, Assertive, Entitled--and More Miserable Than Ever Before* (2014).

Hamilton, D. "Did You Know You're a Chemist?" DrDavidHamilton.com. (2013).

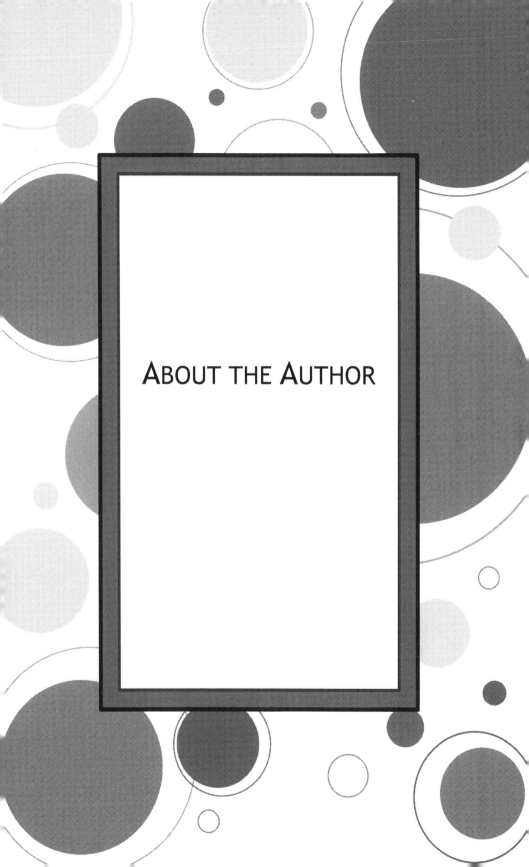

ABOUT THE AUTHOR

About the Author

Dr. Renee Thompson is a sought after speaker, author, consultant, and leading authority on creating healthy workforces by eliminating bullying and incivility. With 25+ years as a clinical nurse, nurse educator, and nurse executive, Renee is an expert on workplace bullying and incivility. She spends the majority of her time working with healthcare organizations that want to cultivate a professional and respectful workforce.

Renee is the CEO of RTConnections and Founder of the Healthy Workforce Institute. She has been repeatedly published, interviewed, and awarded for her work to educate, connect, and inspire current and future nurses. She is the author of several books and travels internationally as a keynote speaker and consultant.

In 2016, Renee received the Nursing Excellence award as a nurse entrepreneur to honor her work to eliminate workplace bullying. She received the first Outstanding Nursing Alumni for Excellence in Leadership Award and Distinguished Alumni recognition from her alma mater. She was a finalist in the Healthcare Heroes Awards as a Healthcare Provider in her hometown of Pittsburgh, PA.

Her blog (HealthyWorkforceInstitute.com/blog/) has won numerous awards as a Top Nursing Blog "must-read" by the online nursing community, and her anti-bullying videos are viewed by healthcare organizations around the world.

Renee is one of only 26 nurses in the world who has achieved the prestigious Certified Speaking Professional (CSP) designation. In 2018, she was recognized as one of LinkedIn's Top Ten Voices in Healthcare for her contribution to their global online healthcare community.

Renee has a master's degree in nursing education and a doctorate of nursing practice from the University of Pittsburgh.

Renee and her husband, Ashley, split their time between Pittsburgh, PA and Tampa, Florida. They are enjoying being new grandparents, making frequent trips to visit little miss Olivia in Raleigh, NC.

To discover more about Renee and how she and her team can help you cultivate a healthy workforce, visit:

Website ....: www.HealthyWorkforceInstitute.com
Email ....: WeCare@RTConnections.com

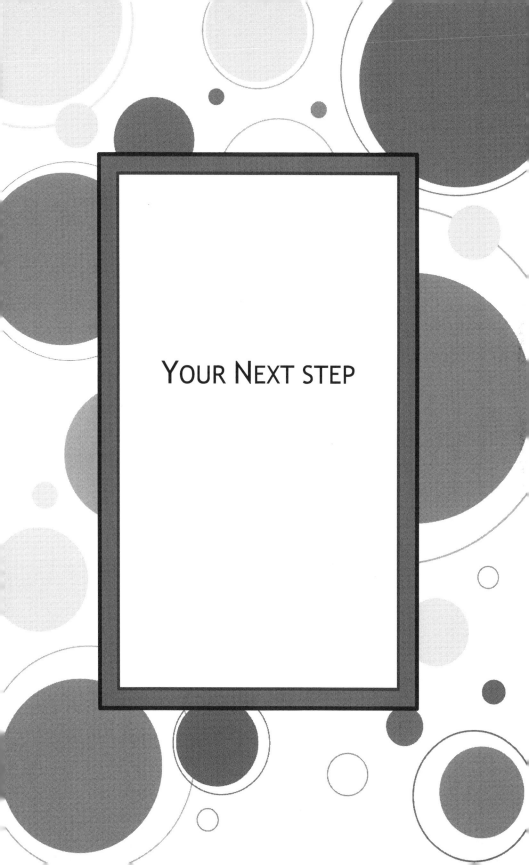

YOUR NEXT STEP

Your Next Step

My intent in writing this book was to give front line leaders the skills and tools they need to address workplace bullying and incivility. However, I'm not a magician. One book may not be enough. For leaders who want to continue their learning and spread these principles across their organization, here are a few options:

Subscribe to My Free Leader Resources

Once a week, I share content specifically designed to help leaders address disruptive behaviors and cultivate a professional workforce culture. My subscribers receive videos, articles, new resources, and a monthly newsletter. Although some of this content is available to the public, some is exclusive just for my subscribers.

Go to https://HealthyWorkforceInstitute.com, to subscribe and enter your name and email address in the box that says, "For Healthcare Leaders."

FOLLOW ME ON SOCIAL MEDIA

I built my business by being active on social media! You can find me on LinkedIn, Facebook, Twitter, and YouTube. I'd love to connect, so feel welcome to follow, like, and subscribe.

LinkedIn........: linkedin.com/in/RTconnections
Facebook ......: facebook.com/RTConnections/
Twitter.........: twitter.com/RTConnections
YouTube ....: youtube.com/c/RTConnections

READ MY BLOG

I've been writing an article about disruptive behaviors in healthcare every week since 2011. Topics include how to build a case with deliberate documentation, how to tell your "best" nurse she's toxic, how to become a better coworker, 10 things every employee wants his or her leader to know, and much more. I offer a mix of articles that swing the pendulum between how to stop the badness and how to cultivate the goodness. My blog has won numerous awards and continues to receive positive attention within the online healthcare community. You'll find it at https://HealthyWorkforceInstitute.com/blog/

ENROLL IN MY COURSE, *ERADICATING BULLYING & INCIVILITY: ESSENTIAL SKILLS FOR HEALTHCARE LEADERS*

As an element of my Healthy Workforce Academy, this course walks a leader through my five-step process for addressing disruptive behaviors. This online course takes leaders down the rabbit hole more than any book can. It helps leaders implement specific strategies and tactics to set behavioral expectations and hold their employees accountable.

However, this is not just any online course! Leaders enrolled in the course receive a 50-minute coaching call with me or a member of my team and have access to a biweekly live Q & A call. This call features additional content, plus the opportunity to ask questions. Participants also receive new resources as we develop them. Leaders can enroll in this course as individuals or as a cohort with other leaders within their organization. To learn more about this course, go to:

https://HealthyWorkforceInstitute.com/programs/eradicating-bullying-incivility-healthcare-leaders/

Or, you can just go to my website:

https://HealthyWorkforceInstitute.com > services > blended learning programs > eradicating bullying and incivility.

INVITE ME TO YOUR ORGANIZATION

I started my business as a speaker. However, because so many organizations wanted more from me, I now offer a cadre of services from books and online courses to keynotes, workshops, and comprehensive consulting. Many times a leader will reach out to me asking for help. That leader knows he or she has a problem with behavior but doesn't know where to begin. One of the most powerful actions organizations can take is to invite me or someone from my team to their organization to heighten awareness through one of our foundational workshops. Once you've heightened awareness, the path toward a healthy workforce culture becomes clear.

If you're interested in finding out how you can bring us to your organization, send us an email with your intent to WeCare@HealthyWorkforceInstitute.com.

Please don't let this book, albeit helpful, be the only resource you invest in. Cultivating and sustaining a healthy workforce culture takes a concerted effort and commitment to continuous learning. Just choose the best option for you!

Made in the USA
Columbia, SC
31 January 2023

11158330R00124